Handbook of

Equine Wound Management

Dedication

This book is dedicated to my two daughters, Clare and Julie, and to my wife Morna. They have tolerated my busy life for many years with good humor, and they are the reason for my existence.

For Saunders:

Commissioning Editor: Joyce Rodenhuis
Senior Development Editor: Zoë A Youd
Project Manager: Gail Wright
Design Direction: Andy Chapman

Handbook of
Equine Wound
Management

Derek C Knottenbelt
BVM&S DVMS DipECEIM MRCVS
Philip Leverhulme Hospital
University of Liverpool
Liverpool, UK

SAUNDERS

SAUNDERS
An imprint of Elsevier Science Limited

First published 2003

ISBN 0 7020 2693 X

British Library Cataloguing in Publication Data
A catalogue record for this book is available from the British Library

Library of Congress Cataloging in Publication Data
A catalog record for this book is available from the Library of Congress

Note
Veterinary knowledge is constantly changing. As new information becomes available, changes
in treatment, procedures, equipment and the use of drugs become necessary. The author and
the publishers have taken great care to ensure that the information given in this text is
accurate and up to date. However, readers are strongly advised to confirm that the
information, especially with regard to drug usage, complies with the latest legislation and
standards of practice.

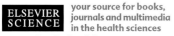
ELSEVIER
SCIENCE

your source for books,
journals and multimedia
in the health sciences
www.elsevierhealth.com

The
publisher's
policy is to use
**paper manufactured
from sustainable forests**

Printed in China by RDC Group Limited

Contents

Contents

Acknowledgements

I am grateful to Professor Barrie Edwards and the staff of the Philip Leverhulme Hospital for their help with clinical cases and advice on wound management.

Drs Christine Cochrane and Jacintha Wilmink have pioneered research into the problems of wound healing in horses and have made equine wound management a new and important area of clinical research. They have contributed much to this booklet and I am truly grateful to them both. Dr Sarah Cockbill and Professor Terry Turner of the Department of Pharmacy, University of Cardiff, have made constructive suggestions and provided useful information for the dressings section.

Thank you also to Professors Barrie Edwards, Dennis Brooks and Jim Schumacher, and Drs Johan Marais, Chris Proudman, Peter Clegg, Ellen Singer, Chris Riggs and Reg Pascoe for providing images, ideas and constructive criticism.

Jonathan Gregory has overseen the production of the booklet with help from Phil Russell of Smith and Nephew. Much of the artwork has been prepared by Gudrun and Adrian Cornford.

Finally, I am grateful to the horses that have provided so much challenge over many years! They have sometimes tolerated their care with fortitude but others have been less cooperative! To them all I say thank you for your contribution to our understanding of wounds and wound management and we hope that future generations will find that their wounds will be managed better and with less pain than their forebears.

I hope that this brief book will be of interest and will generate both an active discussion and further research into the problems of wound healing in horses – a clinical area of study that lags far behind that in the human and other species.

Section 1

Principles and Practice of Equine Wound Management

1 Introduction

The temperament and the type of work it has to perform mean that the horse is probably more prone to accidental injury than most other species. Anatomical knowledge is possibly the most important single aspect of wound management. Many problematic wounds have recognizable anatomical complications that could perhaps have been foreseen at the outset. The wrong treatment, or the right treatment badly executed, can result in the opposite effect to that intended, and may even endanger the animal's life. There remain, however, a proportion of wounds that simply will not heal and these are a major problem in equine practice.

Over the last 10–20 years there have been considerable advances in our understanding of wound healing, and this information is finally reaching the clinical situation for horses. Since 1962, wound dressing technology has played a much more active role in the healing process, and so wounds can reasonably be expected to heal much more efficiently and with much less scar and functional deficit. Dressings can be selected and adjusted for the exact needs of the specific stage of healing in a wound. However, there are no dressings that are suitable for all types of wound and all stages of healing; indeed, there are circumstances when dressings may not be helpful.

Where a wound fails to heal as expected, the clinician should be able to recognize the possible reasons for this in most cases. The horse appears to have particular difficulty with healing, especially in the limb regions of larger horses. Although recently there have been considerable advances, there remains further research to do before we will fully understand the healing process in the horse.

Chapter Preview

▶ Graze/Abrasion/Erosion

▶ Bruising

▶ Hematoma

▶ Contusion

▶ Puncture Wound

▶ Incised Wound

▶ Laceration

▶ Complicated Wound

▶ Burns

2 Definition of Wounds/Wound Types

Although wounds are given specific classifications there are many that have properties of several specific types; indeed there are seldom any classical wounds apart from those afflicted in the course of elective or other surgical procedures.

Graze/Abrasion/Erosion (Figure 1)

A graze is a superficial denuding of the epidermis with minimal (capillary) bleeding and usually some serum/plasma exudation, often in pinpoint form at first. It arises from abrasion against a rough or hard object such as a road surface.

Clinical management of grazes involves application of soothing ointments such as silver sulfadiazine (e.g. Flamazine, Smith and Nephew) to encourage rapid epithelialization and prevent infection. Healing is usually complete, uncomplicated, uneventful, and rapid, and usually there is no visible scar.

Moist wound management methods hasten recovery and reduce pain significantly.

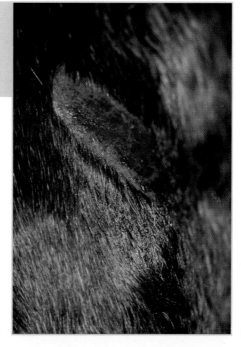

Figure 1 A graze sustained from contact with a concrete floor. The epidermis is stripped but the dermis is not totally disrupted. Healing is usually rapid with negligible scarring.

Bruising (Figure 2)

Bruising is the result of bleeding and tissue destruction within and under the intact skin, that causes damage to capillary beds or larger blood vessels. Bruising can occur in tissue adjacent to a laceration or without any outward injury. It may be difficult to detect skin bruising in horses because of the skin color and dense hair coat. The extent of the bruise is variable, but where multiple significant bruises arise from relatively trivial trauma then clotting parameters should be checked.

Treatment is seldom required, but in some sites (such as eyelids or penis) ice packs or possibly cold-hosing can be used to reduce the local inflammation and control swelling, and minimize further damage to the skin. Healing is usually uneventful and with minimal scarring.

Hematoma (Figure 3)

A hematoma is the accumulation of a large volume of free blood under the skin. Hematoma can be differentiated from edema or inflammatory fluid by the 'finger press test'. In the case of edema, a finger pressed onto the swelling and then removed will leave an indent that remains visible for some minutes. If the swelling is inflammatory, there will probably be no pitting with pressure; in the case of hematoma the indentation will disappear immediately the finger is removed.

Hematoma can be left to organize or can be drained according to clinical preferences. Direct pressure to the drained area is sometimes helpful, but can also be difficult in some locations. A pressure stent sutured over the site or a firm bandage, where this is feasible, may limit extent and shorten recovery.

Healing may be problematical with slow organizing and fibrosis, or continued bleeding or abscessation. The skin may crinkle at the site, or there may be some functional problems if there is extensive fibrosis. A scar may be visible as distorted skin, firmly bound down to the underlying tissues. Organizing hematoma in some sites (e.g. penile skin) can cause functional problems.

Contusion (Figure 4)

Contusions are common; they are in effect severe bruises with some skin injury.

A contusion is rarely a problem, except where it involves structures other than skin. One of the commonest sites for contusions is the head (periorbital region) in horses that have severe colic. The damage around the eyes involves bruising and superficial grazing. Secondary effects include conjunctival edema (with protrusion). Contusions are usually managed by a combination of ice packs and prophylactic antibiotics. Healing is usually uneventful but some permanent scarring can occur.

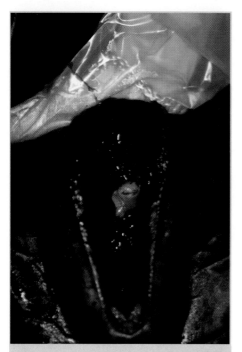

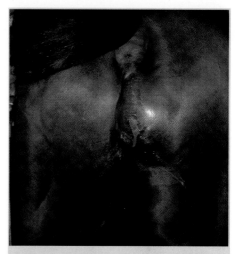

Figure 3 A hematoma resulting from a kick to the perineum of a mare.

Figure 2 Bruising of the vulva during parturition. There is extensive diffuse bleeding into the tissues without a break in the overlying skin.

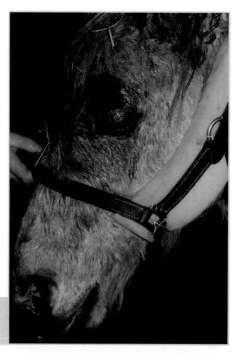

Figure 4 A contusion over the eye sustained as a result of self-inflicted trauma during colic.

Puncture Wound (Figures 5, 6)

Puncture wounds in the skin and hoof from sharp objects (e.g. nails, glass shards, or other foreign bodies) are common and potentially very serious. Puncture wounds may easily be overlooked or trivialized, as the size of the wound often belies the potential severity of the injury; the skin defect is usually trivial by comparison to the deeper damage, which can even be fatal if it affects a vital organ such as the synovial structures of the foot or the cranium, or carries (anaerobic) infection into the wound. This type of wound proves the ideal anaerobic environment for *Clostridium tetani* organisms to flourish.

Infection of the interstitial tissues and the lymphatic vessels is termed cellulitis and lymphangitis, respectively. In either case infection can spread extensively from the site of the injury.

The wounds may be difficult to explore effectively. Puncture wounds must be treated by scrupulous cleaning and, if necessary, widening of the injury to avoid anaerobic conditions. Antibiotics and non-steroidal anti-inflammatory drugs are usually used, but controlled movement is usually considered to be an important aid to treatment. Ice packs and cold-hosing of the affected limb may be helpful.

Healing of the skin wound is incidental and usually uncomplicated in all cases.

Incised Wound (Figure 7)

An incised wound (including a surgical wound) has a sharp defined margin and is caused by sharp metal or glass, flint, or occasionally the leading edge of a shoe. The skin is cut cleanly with minimal tearing and bruising of the wound margins. Injuries may extend into other structures, e.g. tendons and synovial sheaths; these are classified as complicated wounds (see p. 100, Section 3).

Some bleeding is common, although reflex vasospasm limits instant blood loss. Thereafter, there may be considerable hemorrhage associated with vasodilatation, especially if arteries are involved. Hemorrhage may be controlled by pressure bandaging or clamping/ligation of significant vessels (see p. 39). Treatment is straightforward: primary closure by suture, adhesive, or simply by dressings.

Note: Nerves and arteries often run in close proximity, so blindly feeling for the vessel with a pair of hemostats in the conscious horse can be dangerous!

In most cases, healing is rapidly achieved. Scarring is usually obvious but of limited functional importance.

Laceration (Figure 8)

A laceration is a traumatic tearing of the skin in an uncontrolled direction. Lacerated wounds are common, and multiple tears in the skin may be accompanied by bruising. Hemorrhage is rarely a problem.

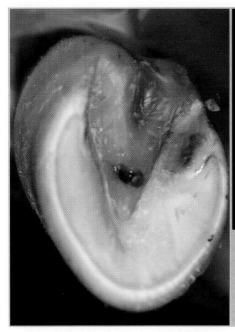

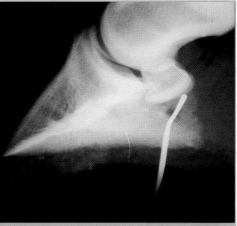

Figures 5, 6 Puncture wound on the sole from a nail penetration (**5**, left), and a radiograph showing the extent of the damage resulting from the nail penetration (**6**, right). This is extremely dangerous.

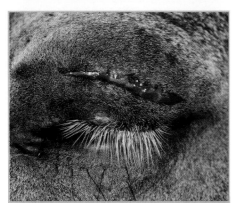

Figure 7 This is an accidental incised wound; there is no complicating deeper damage and the margins are sharply incised. Primary intention healing is to be expected in this case, scarring will be minimal and no functional problems are likely.

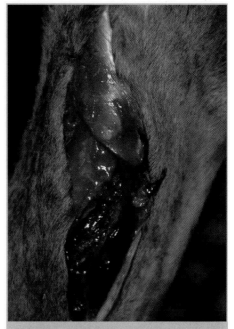

Figure 8 A laceration on the lateral aspect of the hock. Such wounds often have insignificant bleeding. The clot is visible in the wound.

Treatment of lacerations is described in Section 3. Healing is often difficult especially on the limbs. The prognosis is less favorable than for incised wounds because tissue necrosis and sloughing are frequent complications.

Complicated Wound (Figures 9, 10)

Complicated wounds are probably the commonest wound type in equine practice. Injuries either involve other structures or are complicated by factors that either preclude simple primary union, or are likely to result in serious delays in healing.

Involvement of other organs or structures may be more significant than the skin injury itself. Some injuries are life threatening; these wounds are considered in full in Section 3 (see p. 95).

Healing depends on the extent of damage and the ability of structures involved to heal but will inevitably be problematical.

Burns

Burns can be:
1. Thermal burns (Figure 11).
2. Scalding.
3. Friction burns (rope galls or grass grazes).
4. Chemical/caustic and exudate 'burns'.
5. Freeze 'burns'.
6. Actinic/sun burn.

The face and eyes, the breast, back, and legs are most often involved from stable or grass fires. Flash burns from explosions usually affect the head, breast, and neck. Secondary effects such as smoke inhalation, shock, or toxic absorption may be critical. Rope or focal burns from other causes are simply forms of skin necrosis resulting from friction rather than flames.

Burns are described by extent (percentage of body surface) and depth of tissue damage (first, second, and third degree). The true extent of the damage may not be apparent immediately.

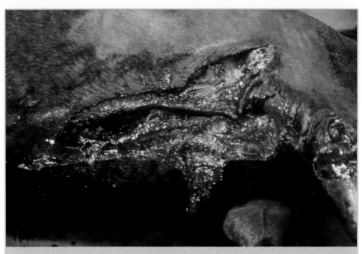

Figure 9 A severe complicated laceration with extensive muscle damage. Note the lack of serious bleeding in spite of the extent of the trauma.

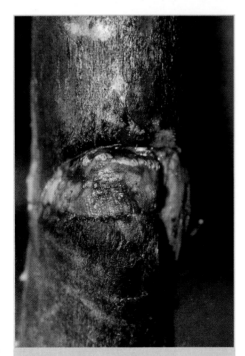

Figure 10 A complicated laceration involving the palmar aspect of the cannon region. There is severe damage and contamination of the superficial and deep flexor tendons.

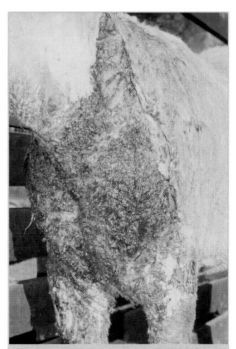

Figure 11 Extensive thermal burn resulting in a large area of severely damaged skin. (Courtesy of RR Pascoe.)

Chapter Preview

3 The Pathophysiology of Wound Healing

Healing

Healing is a complex process that, for descriptive purposes, is arbitrarily divided into three temporally and spatially linked stages (Figure 12):
1. Inflammatory and debridement phase (demarcation).
2. Repair phase (proliferation).
3. Maturation phase (epithelialization and contraction).

Each phase has its local and systemic requirements and will, in turn, influence the others. The clinical objective is to culminate in a closed (healed) wound with a reasonable restoration of both function and cosmesis. The duration of the various phases is variable depending on the site of the wound, the cause of the wound, and the extent of tissue deficits.

Many factors have been identified as having an influence on wound healing; however, any individual factor that adversely (or more rarely beneficially) affects any component of the healing process inevitably carries a penalty (or reward) in the rate and quality of reparative processes (see p. 25).

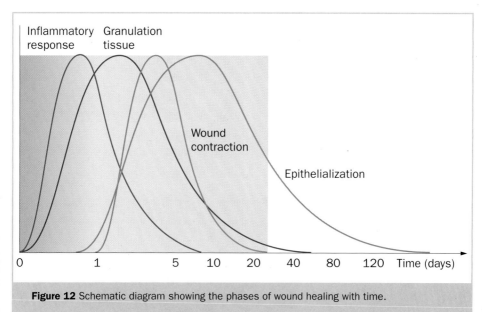

Figure 12 Schematic diagram showing the phases of wound healing with time.

Inflammatory and Debridement (Demarcation) Phase

Blood and fibrin flow into the wound site and form a fibrocellular clot, comprising mainly fibrin and fibronectin with the normal blood cells enmeshed within it (Figure 13). The clot serves to limit blood loss and provides a scaffold for the formation of a new matrix that will facilitate the migration of cells. The migration of phagocytic cells is vital for the natural debridement of the wound (Figure 14). Foreign matter and bacteria are removed, and non-viable tissue is demarcated and gradually separated from the viable areas.

Repair (Proliferative/Granulation) Phase

This usually commences in the first 12 hours; however, it cannot proceed until any remaining blood clots, necrotic tissue debris, and infection have been eliminated. The process cannot proceed without a good blood supply; angiogenesis is critical to the health of the wound.

Healthy sutured wounds are normally covered in 12–24 hours. Full thickness wounds only epithelialize after formation of a granulating bed, necessitating a lag phase of 4–5 days (Figure 15). Migration of fibroblasts and fibroplasia results in a major gain in tensile strength at 5–15 days in the sutured wound. Granulation tissue comprising of a loose extracellular matrix and increasing numbers of fibroblasts and vascular elements begins to develop 3–6 days postinjury and continues until epithelialization occurs (Figure 16).

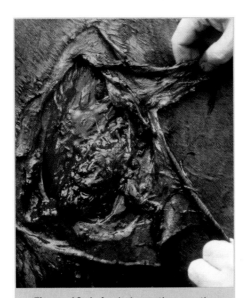

Figure 13 A fresh laceration on the shoulder of a racehorse showing tissue damage. This represents the earliest stages of the acute inflammatory response with clot formation.

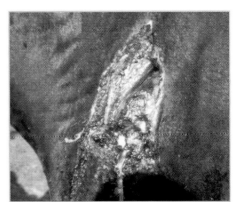

Figure 14 This extensive wound is undergoing natural debridement. Note contraction of the wound.

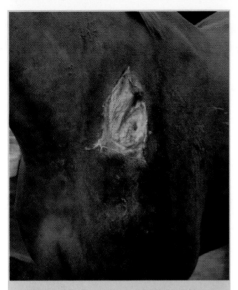

Figure 15 The mid repair phase. Note the advancing epithelial margin and the central red granulation tissue bed.

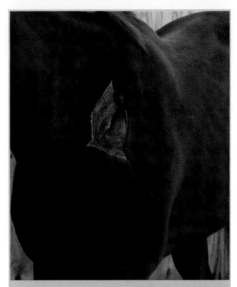

Figure 16 Late repair phase with a healthy epithelial margin and a flat pale granulation tissue bed.

Granulation Tissue

Granulation tissue (Figure 17) is a complex of fibroblasts, vascular endothelial cells (with neovascularization), and macrophages within a collagen and fibrin matrix.
Granulation tissue:
1. Provides a surface for epithelialization.
2. Is resistant to infection.
3. Is necessary for wound contraction.

The horse has a particular propensity for the formation of exuberant granulation tissue at wound sites on the limb. This problem does not appear to affect ponies at all, nor wound sites on the body trunk and neck/head of larger horses unless there are defined reasons for the failure of healing (see Section 2, p.25).

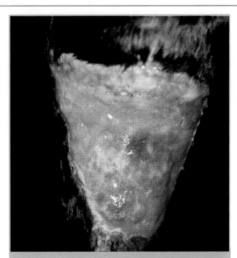

Figure 17 A healthy bed of granulation tissue on the dorsal hock region. There is little evidence of marginal epithelial ingrowth or wound contraction.

Maturation Phase (Epithelialization and Contraction) (Figures 18, 19)

Epithelialization is a very slow process in which the keratinocytes migrate centripetally. It starts within hours of wounding, but on the limbs proceeds at a maximum rate of around 1–1.5 mm/10 days. The healing edge of a limb wound may only be visible after 10–14 days. Epithelialization is retarded by the presence of fibrin clot in the wound, and also by the products of chronic inflammation and death of polymorphonuclear leukocytes.

The healing epithelium is fragile and thin and is poorly adherent to the underlying tissues. As the epithelium is restored and the underlying fibrous tissue and granulation tissue is remodeled, a scar is formed. Tension applied to the wound initiates scar strengthening along lines of force within the healing tissue. The scar regains only 80% of the original tissue tensile strength at 1 year; the new collagen is of a different type, which lacks the cross-links of 'normal' collagen. The scar gradually shrinks with decreasing vascularity and cellularity until eventually it is comprised mainly of dense fibrocytes.

The Healing Process

Full restoration of natural anatomy is seldom if ever achieved. Scarring is the inevitable outcome of wounding in any tissue. In some cases this limits function or the cosmetic appearance.

Healing can be achieved in one of three ways:
1. Primary or first intention healing.
2. Secondary or second intention healing.
3. Delayed primary healing

Primary (First Intention) Healing (Figure 20)

This is usually used where suturing easily reunites wound margins, and there is no detectable reason for wound healing failure. Minimal granulation tissue formation and epithelial migration are required. Few accidental wounds are amenable to this approach (Table 1). In a non-infected surgical wound, healing is reliably accomplished in a predictably short time.

Table 1 The major mechanisms of healing applicable to surgical and accidental wounds	
Surgical wound	Accidental wound
First intention healing:	Second intention healing:
Rapid healing	Slow healing
Small scar	Extensive scarring
Rapid restoration of tissue strength	Slow/weak tissue strength
Minimal infection/complication	Complication rate high

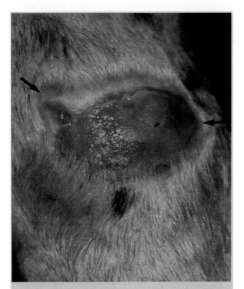

Figure 18 A partially healed wound showing an epithelial margin and evidence of contraction (note the contraction lines, arrows).

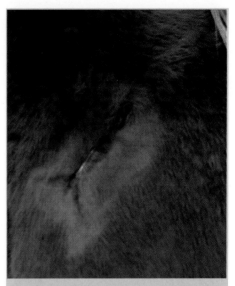

Figure 19 A mature wound with a scar that is much smaller than the original wound (see Figures 13–16). The skin is not normal, but is a satisfactory replacement (cosmesis is good).

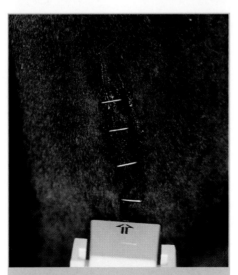

Figure 20 A simple incised wound over the lateral aspect of the distal cannon that is expected to heal by primary union after being closed by staples. The wound healed without complication or significant scar.

Elective surgical wounds are probably the current 'gold standard' of wound management but there are major differences between surgical wounds and accidental injuries (see Table 2), and so there are almost inevitable differences in healing.

Second Intention Healing

In second intention healing granulation tissue must fill the base of the wound before epithelialization can be completed (Figure 21). This inevitably extends the time required for healing. Wounds too extensive or contaminated to suture, or those in which primary closure has failed, must heal in this way (Figures 22–24).

Second intention healing relies upon the inflammatory response; the longer the wound takes to heal the greater will be the scar and the possible cosmetic and functional deficits. The problems associated with second intention healing may encourage clinicians to try to close wounds by primary union even although this can be both difficult and disappointing.

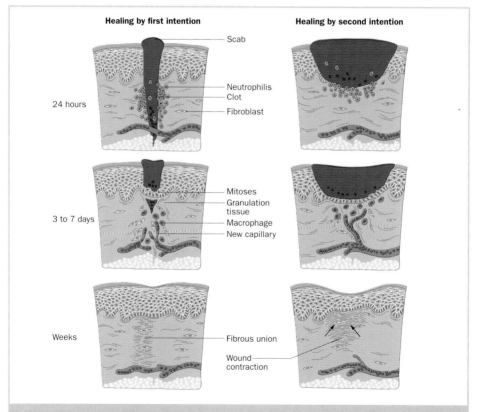

Figure 21 Steps in wound healing by first intention (left) and second intention (right). In the latter, the resultant scar is smaller than the original wound, owing to wound contraction, but is still larger than an equivalent primary healed wound.

Table 2 The major clinically important differences between surgical wounds and accidental wounds

Surgical Wounds	Accidental wound
Predictable site	Unpredictable site
Predictable direction	Unpredictable direction
Predictable tissue involvement	Unpredictable tissue involvement
Minimal skin damage	Concurrent bruising and tearing of skin
Closure by primary union is the norm	Closure by primary union is less usual and may be difficult
Wound break down is rare	Wound break down is relatively frequent
Infection is preventable and is rarely significant	Infection is an almost inevitable complication and is common

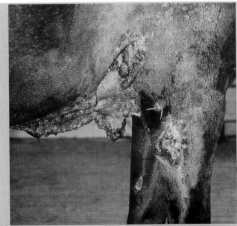

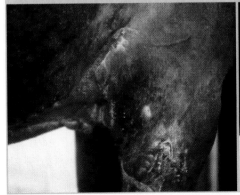

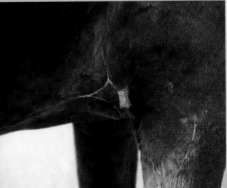

Figures 22–24 Photo series of healing by second intention (the initial wound is shown in Figure 9). This series shows (**22**) a large lacerated wound in the axilla, brisket and girth region that (**23**) healed well with significant contraction by day 32, and (**24**) by day 90 has almost resolved completely by contraction rather than epithelialization. The epithelial expansion was 0.8–1.3 cm wide at its widest points.

Second intention healing occurs faster in ponies than in horses and body wounds heal faster than limb wounds[1]. Over 70% of equine limb wounds are complicated by failure to heal and chronic inflammation. The reasons for this focus on the inflammatory response, which is more intense and of shorter duration in ponies than in horses. The myofibroblasts are better arranged to result in contraction in the smaller equidae[2].

Delayed Primary Union Healing (Figures 25, 26)

This is a combination of the early stages of second intention healing with a final primary intention healing after a few days. It is a useful procedure in many contaminated wounds in which immediate closure may lead to complication. If closure is delayed for 72–96 hours, only a minimal risk of infection exists. The wound is cleaned and debrided but is not closed. After a variable time (usually 2–4 days) the wound is surgically debrided and closed by suture as for first intention healing.

The clinical advantages of delayed primary healing are considerable:
1. The wound can be assessed for causes of failure of healing at various stages allowing the best time for closure to be chosen.
2. Acute inflammatory responses and natural debridement can take place before it is 'driven' towards healing without the development of a difficult and prolonged chronic inflammatory process.

Problems relate to delays in healing and the need for repeated procedures. Furthermore, there is an inevitable increase in scarring when compared to first intention healing, although the time delay may be relatively insignificant.

Wound Contraction

Contraction is the process whereby intact skin bordering on a full thickness skin deficit is drawn in centripetally over the wound bed in the early stages of repair.

Wound contraction is the result of a higher centripetal force at the wound margins than the centrifugal forces of skin contraction and shrinkage (see Figures 19 and 22). It is the major factor in the closure/healing of body trunk or neck wounds in horses.

There are significant differences in wound contraction between different sites on the body and between horses and ponies[3]; wound contraction is greater in ponies than in horses, and is more efficient and pronounced in body wounds than in limb wounds. Significant contraction does not usually occur below the carpus and hock. Many wounds on the distal limb of larger horses (over 140 cm) fail to heal, and the wound often appears to become larger, i.e. the centrifugal forces exceed the centripetal ones.

Wound contraction commences after a lag phase of approximately 6–8 days and in small wounds is complete in 10–12 days. In large wounds it may not be complete for several weeks. Contraction of wounds healing by primary union is insignificant, but is most important in wounds that are allowed to heal by second intention. Up to 70% of the skin deficit may be eliminated in this way, the remainder being achieved by epithelialization.

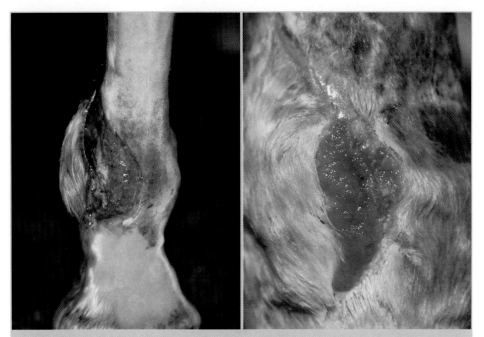

Figures 25, 26 A laceration over the lateral fetlock region that was first presented some 24 hours after injury. The wound was managed by delayed primary union. The sutures were placed over most of the length of the wound 4 days after presentation, following two surgical debridement procedures. The distal part could not be closed due to skin contraction and some skin necrosis.

The mechanism depends upon the conversion of fibroblasts into myofibroblasts by the inclusion of smooth muscle actin (SMA) into the fibroblasts[4], instigated by transforming growth factor-beta (TGF-β)[5]. The increased tendency to contraction in ponies may be explained at least in part by the much higher concentrations of TGF-β in the granulation tissue. The variations are due to local factors rather than any inherent differences in the cells themselves.

Note

Wound contraction can be viewed as a considerable ally in the repair of body wounds in horses. In some species however, such as man in particular, contraction is frequently a serious disadvantage. Many wounds in man continue to contract long after the wound has closed and this can result in serious functional limitations.

Section 2
Healing Delay

Chapter Preview

▶ Infection/Infestation

▶ Movement

▶ Foreign Body

▶ Necrotic Tissue

▶ Altered Local pH

▶ Paucity of Blood Supply

▶ Poor (or Impaired) Oxygen Supply

▶ Poor Nutritional and Health Status

▶ Local Factors

▶ Iatrogenic Factors

▶ Genetic Factors

▶ Cell Transformation

4 Factors that Delay Healing

Factors that disturb normal corrective processes inevitably complicate wound healing. Early recognition of healing difficulties allows prompt correction. Delayed healing inevitably results in development of chronic inflammation, and although transition through the chronic inflammatory stage is almost inevitable in naturally occurring wounds, it is the most undesirable event in the healing cascade.

Prolonged chronic inflammation causes progressive production of exuberant granulation tissue, or alternatively a reduction in the production of granulation tissue; in either case, an inhibited epithelial cell replication results.

The longer a wound takes to heal the larger will be the scar and the longer will be the recovery period. The more extensive the scar the greater may be the limitations to function. Most non-healing wounds are preventable by suitable management in the early stages after injury, and others are understandable or predictable. Failure to recognize potential reasons for failure of healing means that the wound will become chronically inflamed and so the healing process will be unnecessarily prolonged. Healing failure mediated through chronic inflammation can be instigated by several factors described below.

Infection/Infestation

Infected wounds heal slower than uninfected ones. Mixed infections are relatively common (Figure 27), and tissue bacteria numbers above 1×10^6 organisms delays healing[6]. Bacterial species that produce collagenase or other destructive enzymes have a profound effect on healing (Figure 28).

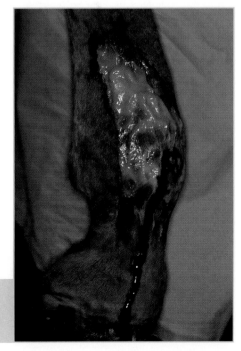

Figure 27 An infected granulating wound on the distal cannon. A mixed growth of bacteria was cultured.

Infection with *Staphylococcus aureus* can cause pyogranuloma within the wound site. Clinically this resembles both granulation tissue and sarcoid, but histologically diffuse microabscessation is present (Figure 29).

Fungal infections of superficial wounds is relatively common. For example, *Pythius* spp., or *Basidiobolus haptosporus* infection (deep or superficial mycosis or hyphomycosis) can be catastrophic complications of relatively trivial wounds. Parasitic infestation, e.g. with *Habronema musca* or the larvae of certain flies (myiasis), also retards healing (Figure 30). The larvae of *Lucilla sericata* has been found to have a beneficial debriding effect in some wounds under controlled conditions.

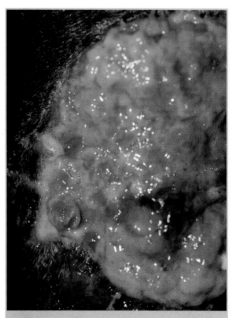

Figure 28 A severely infected non-healing wound from which a pure growth of *Pseudomonas aeruginosa* was cultured.

Movement

Movement at the site or in the attached tissues delays healing (Figure 31). Excessive mobility disrupts capillary buds and increases collagen deposition, directing the healing process towards chronic inflammatory status. Anatomical knowledge may establish the likelihood of deep tissues that are moving significantly relative to the wound itself. Wounds on the body may fail to heal because of movement of the underlying muscle, but this is less significant in horses.

Movement at the site or in the attached tissues, e.g. flexor tendon in the palmar cannon area results in marked disruptive forces within the wound. Lack of all movement can also be counter-productive to strong healing, due to the lack of arrangement of collagen along stress lines.

Foreign Body

Foreign bodies are one of the commonest reasons for non-healing wounds, and include foreign matter (e.g. sand or grit particles, wood or other plant matter, or metal/glass) or necrotic tissue (e.g. bone, tendon, skin). Hair can be driven into the wound or can be deposited during wound clipping.

Some foreign matter will eventually decay or be removed by phagocytes but some will not. Suture materials are also foreign bodies but modern monofilament and absorbable synthetic materials are far less liable to affect healing than many of the older ones (Figure 32). Some foreign bodies are encapsulated in a dense fibrous capsule and then become effectively inert.

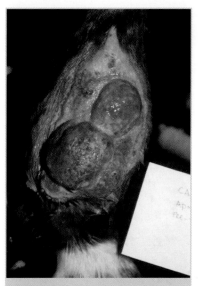

Figure 29 This wound failed to heal because of staphylococcal microabscessation (pseudomyce-toma/botriomycosis).

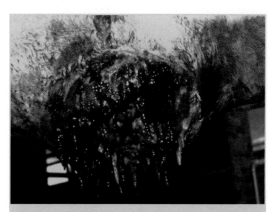

Figure 30 *Habronema musca* infestation of wound on the ventral abdomen, illustrating the role of parasitic infestation in inhibition of wound healing. (Courtesy of J Marais.)

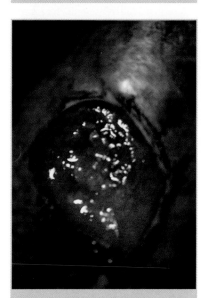

Figure 31 This wound failed to heal because of movement of the damaged common extensor tendon. Movement of joints also causes delays in healing.

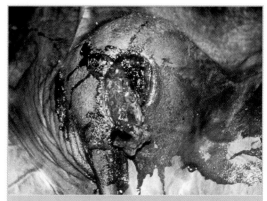

Figure 32 This surgical castration wound failed to heal over 18 months because the cord had been ligated with a piece of ordinary cotton string.

Necrotic Tissue

Necrotic/devitalized tissue of any type (including skin, connective tissue, muscle, tendon, or bone) retards healing significantly. Tendon and bone are often slow to exhibit patent non-viability, and so it may be some months before the necrotic tissue is obvious. It is often wise to allow the natural demarcation of non-viable tissue to be come apparent before wounds are closed (see Delayed Primary Union Healing, p.20). In some cases development of necrotic tissue can be delayed and recognition of this is an important aspect of client management.

Careful debridement of all non-viable tissue at the initial stages of a wound produces a significant benefit (Figure 33).

Altered Local pH

Certain bacteria will induce a highly acid site, while others will induce an alkaline site. The ideal circumstance should be around normal physiological pH or very slightly acidic.

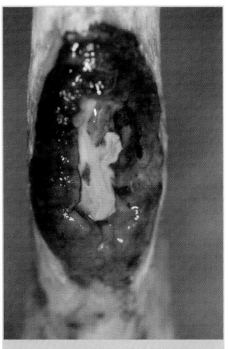

Figure 33 This wound to the palmar aspect of the cannon failed to heal because of unhealthy and necrotic tendon tissue. Once this was removed it healed well, although it was still protracted.

Paucity of Blood Supply

The regional blood supply may be impaired as a result of:
1. Major vessel disruption (gangrene is a manifestation of this).
2. Thrombosis, edema, or contusion.
3. Damage to the microcirculation from ischemia (or even the limited duration vasoconstriction caused by adrenaline included in local anesthetic agents).
4. Anemia (heavy blood loss and conditions associated with serious anemia) is capable of retarding healing significantly (see p. 125).
5. Delay in capillary formation.

Some areas of the horse's skin such as the dorsal hock region are thought to have a naturally poorer blood supply than other areas.

Poor (or Impaired) Oxygen Supply

Adequate oxygenation is important for normal healing; lowered systemic oxygenation due to decreased blood flow in microcirculation slows wound healing and encourages the development of chronic inflammation. Low surface oxygen tension can, however, also stimulate angiogenesis.

Mild anemia does not itself have much influence, but profound anemia will cause low local oxygen tension. The cause of the anemia may be more important than the low red cell volume itself. Anaerobic conditions in a wound can be conducive to the development of some of the most serious clostridial infections.

Modern gas permeable dressings enhance the oxygen gradient and surface carbon dioxide tension and so improve healing.

Poor Nutritional and Health Status

Debilitated and/or old horses heal more slowly than healthy young ones.

Hypoalbuminemia (serum albumin below 30 g/L) significantly retards healing and encourages chronic inflammation. Vitamin A and C deficiency can retard healing; it is unlikely that horses on normal diets will be deficient in these.

Clinically significant loss of zinc can occur from exudative open wounds and can cause delay in healing. Affected wounds are often 'jelly-like' with poor granulation tissue quality and little or no epithelialization.

> ## Note
>
> **Equine Cushing's disease cases commonly heal badly because of the high circulating cortisone concentrations. A horse with significant anemia and/or hypoproteinemia as a result of a wound can lose weight and the wound may fail to heal. This chronic cycle can be a really important aspect of wound management, and emphasizes the need to perform a thorough clinical (physical) examination of all cases.**

Local Factors

Wounds with a pouch of skin, which cannot drain effectively, and excessive dead space fail to heal. The accumulated fluid may be an ideal medium for bacterial replication. Self-trauma is unusual but occasional wounds seem to irritate or annoy the patient; sometimes a dressing (or cast) is resented rather than the wound itself. Wounds with parasitic infestation may be irritating.

Iatrogenic Factors

Incision, swabbing, hemostasis by forceps, ligature or electrocoagulation, the use of retractors, and sutures are all variously injurious to tissue. Sutures can act as foreign bodies, but new materials have fewer problems. Adverse reactions to sutures can be minimized by using:
1. The finest gauge capable of coapting the tissues
2. Atraumatic needles.
3. An appropriate suture pattern.
4. The least amount of suture material possible.

Excessive pressure from dressings can compromise blood supply and the surface oxygen tension. Pressure is sometimes used to control or prevent exuberant granulation tissue but this must be done very carefully. Strong or weak acids or caustic chemicals, such as silver nitrate, potassium permanganate, or copper sulfate damage tissue repair mechanisms.

Note

All physiologically unsound materials are completely unacceptable in normal wound management practice.

Corticosteroids suppress:
1. Acute and chronic inflammatory stages.
2. Angiogenesis.
3. Fibroplasia.
4. Wound contraction[7].

Note

The importance of the acute inflammatory response cannot be overemphasized.
Corticosteroids should not be applied to recent/fresh wounds although a single dose of fast acting cortisone is unlikely to have any material effect on healing. Exogenous cortisone may encourage infection by suppression of macrophage and neutrophil activity. Corticosteroids can be beneficial in reducing or controlling chronic inflammatory responses, and are a useful management tool (see p. 87).

Genetic Factors

Individual horses (and genetic lines) heal less well than others. Larger horses heal less efficiently than ponies, especially in the distal limb regions. Horses with congenitally weakened skin (e.g. hyperelastosis cutis/Ehlers–Danlos syndrome) have fragile skin that is more easily traumatized than normal, and wound healing may be very protracted.

Cell Transformation

This is usually in the form of sarcoid transformation which occurs at wound sites[8, 9]. Healing is inhibited until all tumor cells are removed. Body trunk or facial wounds that contain sarcoid cells usually develop verrucose sarcoid, while limb wounds develop fibroblastic sarcoid (Figure 34).

Sarcoid lesions at other sites, or sarcoids on 'in-contact' horses, predispose tumor transformation. Flies may be involved in sarcoid transformation.

Note

Wounds on horses with sarcoids at other sites should be treated particularly carefully, no matter how small and insignificant the wound appears to be.

Some wounds will partially heal, while others fail to heal at all even if the overall extent of sarcoid involvement is small. The diagnosis of sarcoid transformation requires multiple biopsies. If sarcoid tissue is present, grafts will not take.

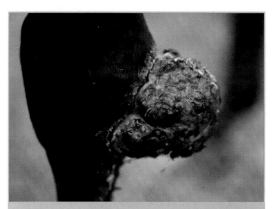

Figure 34 A large fibroblastic sarcoid that developed at the site of a relatively trivial wound on the lateral carpal region. The horse had several other sarcoids.

Section 3
Wound Management

Chapter Preview

► Owner Protocol for Wound Management

► Protocol for Veterinary Attention

► Minimizing the Potential Problems of a Wound

5 General Principles of Wound Managment

Owner Protocol for Wound Management (Figure 35)

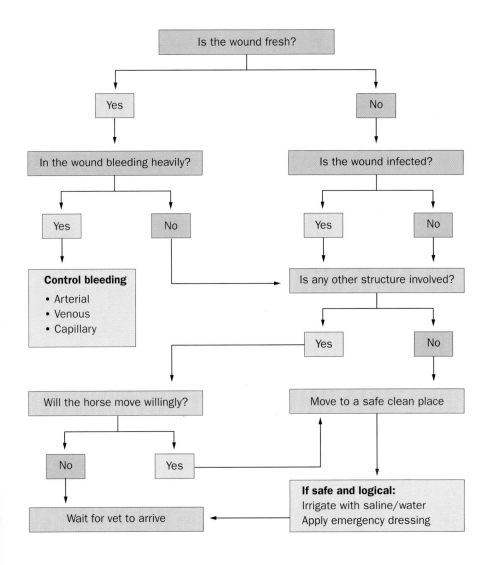

Protocol for Veterinary Attention (Figure 36)

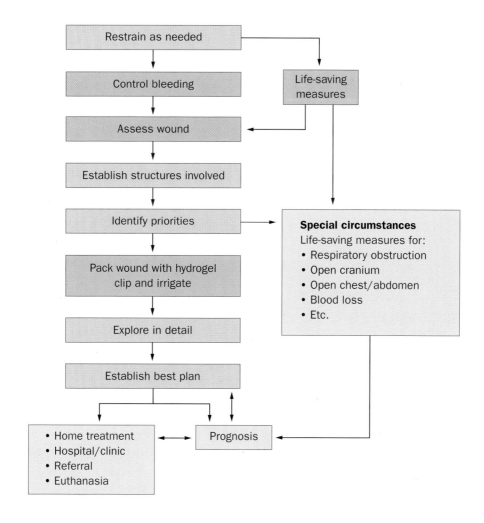

Minimizing the Potential Problems of a Wound

'Time spent in the preparation of a wound is never wasted.'
Barrie Edwards, 1984.

Wound healing is dependent upon fine interactions between the healing elements; it is most unlikely that any single therapy will stimulate the entire normal healing process. Harmful effects can be minimized by careful wound preparation and sound surgical techniques including:

1. Early intervention: bacterial adhesion occurs around 4–8 hours after wounding and therefore intervention before this occurs provides a much cleaner wound. Long delays in attention to a wound inevitably result in overt infection and contamination by foreign matter. Delay in wound examination may however, make recognition of non-viable tissue easier.
2. The application of sound surgical principles.
3. The use of appropriate debridement techniques.
4. The use of suitably placed surgical drains (vacuum drains and Penrose [capillary] drains).
5. Minimizing dead space.
6. Reducing and controlling infection.
7. Eliminating and preventing contamination.
8. The use of physiologically sound wound lavage mechanisms (see p. 46).

Summary

Recognition of potential problems (factors that might be responsible for wound healing) (see p. 25) allows decisions on the best and most appropriate management and the likely course of healing. Consideration of the problems from the outset will almost always result in earlier and more satisfactory healing. By the nature of their location and severity many wounds will have particular limitations and needs and these must be addressed from the outset of wound management.

Chapter Preview

6 Basic Wound Management

After any emergency treatment, such as arresting serious hemorrhage, the horse should, if possible, be moved to a more suitable environment for assessment and treatment. All wounds must be promptly and thoroughly examined to determine the exact site, depth and direction of the wound, and which anatomical tissues and structures are involved and to what extent. It is essential to determine whether important structures, e.g. joints, tendons, nerves, or blood vessels have been damaged. The risk of complications may thereby be minimized and the owner appraised of possible complications in healing at the outset of treatment.

History

The cause and time of the injury should be determined; sometimes they can only be surmised. The cause of the wound and the time delay between injury and veterinary attention will have important implications for the subsequent management.

Tetanus status should always be determined and appropriate protection ensured.

Horses that are receiving drugs for other purposes may have healing problems (either from the underlying disease or from the drugs themselves).

Restraint

Sedatives, opioid analgesic drugs with non-steroidal anti-inflammatory drugs make initial assessment far easier. Suitable drug doses for initial wound management are available.

Initial Examination

Hemorrhage Control

Arterial Bleeding

This is bright red and under high pressure. Even small arteries can produce significant blood loss. Control of arterial bleeding is effected by either direct pressure over the site (or in the arterial tree on the heart side of the injury) which may need to be maintained for up to 10–15 minutes, or a pressure bandage of a suitable type and shape applied over the site. A wound hydrogel (e.g. Intrasite Gel; Smith and Nephew) and a suitable cushioning dressing (e.g. Allevyn pad or an Allevyn Cavity or an Intrasite Conformable roll; Smith and Nephew) is effective, with a firm secondary layer of a soft cotton bandage (e.g. Soffban; Smith and Nephew) followed by a very firm cotton bandage.

> ## Note
>
> **Pressure bandages can be catastrophic without correct bandaging technique. It may stop the bleeding but leave the horse with extensive skin necrosis or even worse, tendon necrosis. Pressure bandages should not be left on for more than 1–2 hours. Removal of the dressing can reinstigate the bleeding.**

Direct ligation or clamping of the artery can also be used to control arterial bleeding, but direct clamping of the artery with artery forceps (hemostats) can be dangerous particularly on the limbs where the artery and the nerve are in close proximity. *The nerve may not be visible if bleeding is heavy*. Ligation with suture material is a standard technique in surgery but the nerve must not be incorporated in the hemostat or the ligature. Finally, adrenaline swabs can be effective in causing rapid (if temporary) vasoconstriction.

Venous Bleeding

This is usually slower (although it can involve large volumes of blood if a large vein is damaged), and the blood is usually dark red/purple in color. The flow is not under sufficient pressure to squirt from the wound. Venous bleeding can be controlled by direct pressure with a saline soaked swab for a few minutes, application of a firm bandage (a tight 'pressure' bandage is not necessary in most cases), or natural hemostasis, which will usually result in clotting and cessation of bleeding within 10–15 minutes (unless there are clotting problems, the vessel is large, or the venous blood pressure is high).

Capillary Bleeding

This is slow and in small volume but can be either bright or dark in color. Capillary bleeding can be controlled by natural hemostasis (which usually results in cessation of bleeding within a few minutes, but serum may continue to ooze from the site for some hours), cold compresses/ice packs which will result in capillary constriction, or dressings applied to the surface of the wound (particularly alginate dressings).

Initial Cleaning

Time spent in wound preparation is never wasted, and failure to prepare the wound correctly or fully is a common cause of failed/delayed healing. Ideally washing the wound with sterile saline under minimal pressure is best but (warm) running water is commonly used until any gross contamination is dislodged. The final wash should be with normal saline to restore physiological status. Care should be taken to ensure that this does not drive foreign matter into the depths of the wound. If the wound has bled heavily, washing may loosen the blood clot and restart hemorrhage, which may then need to be controlled (see p. 125).

Before clipping, the wound should be packed with a hydrogel or an inert, water-soluble jelly (K-Y Jelly; Johnson and Johnson). After initial clipping and cleaning of the surrounding skin, the hydrogel can be irrigated out of the wound using warm sterile saline under mild pressure (3–5 psi). A solution of 0.5% chlorhexidine is a standard wound antiseptic with minimal harmful effects and can be used if the wound is heavily contaminated or is over 2–4 hours old. Fresh wounds probably do not need an antiseptic wash. Flaps of skin should be lifted and irrigated carefully.

Sterile saline under increased pressure (7–10 psi) is then used. Simply using a 50 ml syringe and squirting the saline directly from it with moderate pressure can achieve this pressure. High pressure can drive bacteria and particles into the tissues and open fascial planes. However, low pressure may fail to dislodge foreign matter and bacteria.

Note

Wiping the wound with dry or saline soaked swabs may just push bacteria and foreign matter deeper into the wound. Strong chemical disinfectants and antiseptics should not be used without considerable thought on the possible balance between benefit and harm (see p. 46).

Wound Assessment

The wound may require local analgesia for full exploration, and suitable agents and sites for regional blocks are available. Regional anesthesia is preferable to local injection as the drugs are invariably acidic and often contain adrenaline.

The wound should be carefully flushed again with warm saline irrigation. Using sterile gloves the wound should be explored digitally to establish the:
1. Depth of the wound.
2. The direction of the damage.
3. The extent of the damage.
4. The precise tissues and structures involved.

Note

The use of a finger is recommended because of the sensitivity with which the wound can be examined. Occasionally the wound is too large to be assessed under local or regional anesthesia, and general anesthesia is preferred.

Prevention of Further Injury and Contamination

Pending a decision for further management it may be helpful to provide a temporary protective antibacterial dressing. A hydrogel is packed into the wound and a suitable protective dressing applied, taking care not to cause further damage.

Infection Control

Up to 6–8 hours after injury, a wound is usually considered *contaminated*. Beyond 6–8 hours, bacteria have usually become established in the damaged tissues and the wound is then classified as *infected*.

Although the so called 'golden period' of up to 6–8 hours after injury is an important concept, it suffers from being too prescriptive. In some cases the wound may be slower or faster to become infected. The overriding principle of wound management is that the wound should be dealt with as soon as possible after injury, and that meticulous assessment and appropriate management support the healing process.

There is merit in administering a full dose of antibiotic before any interference is undertaken; the wound site should be covered throughout the procedure. Topical antibiotics are probably not helpful but sometimes-soluble antibiotic is usefully added to lavage solutions (especially in special or complicated wounds such as wounds involving joints and body cavities).

Factors that Might Retard or Prevent Healing

The presence of any of the recognized factors that might hinder, delay, or prevent healing must be recognized early. Where delayed healing is unavoidable, the owner can be advised accordingly.

Wound Debridement

All foreign matter and necrotic/non-viable tissue should be removed to convert an accidental wound into a surgical one that can be closed by first intention. Debridement is best achieved using a scalpel and dissecting forceps. Extensive debridement may require general anesthesia. Debridement of contaminated/devitalized tissue should be accomplished systematically, starting at the most dependent part of the wound so that bleeding does not conceal tissue that should be removed. Debridement with scissors crushes tissue and so a scalpel should be used for sharp debridement.

In anatomical sites that have little 'spare' skin (e.g. the distal limb regions and the face), or where skin deficits are likely to have serious limiting effects (e.g. the eyelid), skin should be preserved as far as possible. Repeated partial debridement can be performed to produce a clean, healthy wound site.

Surgical debridement may be delayed until it is possible to differentiate between viable and devitalized tissue.

The inability to create a completely sterile wound by debridement and lavage can be partially (but *not* totally) compensated for by:
1. Antibiotics locally and systemically.
2. Provision of adequate drainage.

3. *Partial* suturing.
4. Counter incisions to reduce fluid and tension at the wound site.
5. The use of drains.

Provision of a Moist Environment

A moist wound healing environment has become standard practice. Wounds heal better when maintained in this fashion[10]. Hydrogels, hydrocolloids, and collagen dressings support a moist environment. Hydrophilic, gas permeable, waterproof polymeric foam dressings should be used in the initial stages of wound management. These foams are available in various shapes to allow cavity management. Alginate or highly absorptive dressings may be required if exudate is excessive.

Wound Closure

Primary Closure

Incised wounds (see p. 8) frequently lend themselves to suturing. Suturing should only be carried out when so doing will have a positive advantage and minimal harmful effects. Careful selection of suture patterns will make a considerable difference to wound healing. The standard patterns and their advantages and disadvantages are described on p.48 and in standard surgical texts. No wound should be completely closed unless the deeper tissues are effectively sterile.

Factors that are likely to result in wound breakdown (dehiscence) after suturing include:
1. Gross contamination.
2. Infection.
3. Significant skin loss/tension in suture line
4. Marked swelling.

Note

Delays in closure may result in primary contraction of the skin flaps that may preclude closure. Primary closure will almost always fail when tissue necrosis and swelling disrupt the suture line.

Notwithstanding the presence of obvious complication factors, wounds involving the lower parts of the limbs usually present the greatest challenges. There is considerable controversy over the necessity to suture lower limb wounds. In general, a limb wound may be sutured if the wound is clean, free of complicating factors, and in the longitudinal plane (i.e. running up-down the limb). If the wound is not in a suitable site that makes suturing without undue tension feasible, then it is probably best to use second intention healing (see p. 18) or delayed primary intention healing (see p. 20).

Delayed Primary Closure

This is used in relatively clean but contaminated wounds with extensive tissue damage. The wound is cleaned, debrided and dressed with a hydrogel (Intrasite Gel or Intrasite Conformable; Smith and Nephew), and a polymeric foam dressing (e.g. Allevyn, Smith and Nephew) applied. Cavity dressings (Allevyn Cavity or Intrasite Conformable; Smith and Nephew) or shaped dressings (e.g. Allevyn Heel; Smith and Nephew) can be used in awkward sites.

Reexamination and redressing continues at appropriate intervals until the wound is free of obvious infection and necrotic tissue, and the wound bed contains healthy granulation tissue. The wound is then freshened using careful superficial sharp debridement and closed using a suitable suture technique (possibly with tension relieving quills or tension relieving lateral incisions).

Second Intention Healing

The wound is left open after initial treatment and allowed to granulate. Healthy granulation tissue fills the wound from its depth, and once it reaches the wound margin the epithelium should be able to migrate across the wound. Wound contraction is a significant aspect of second intention healing. It occurs at a rapid rate and is responsible for over 95% of second intention healing on the body and neck.

Contraction is very weak in the distal limb regions of horses in particular (see p. 20). Second intention healing is faster in ponies than in horses, and faster on the body trunk than on the limbs where, at least in a proportion of larger horses, the inflammatory process is weak and prolonged and so the wound never heals[11].

Note

In most horses over 140 cm in height there is no significant contraction in limb wounds, i.e. below the stifle and the elbow, and in particular below the knee (carpus) and the hock (tarsus).

Antibacterial Support

Failure to control potential and actual infection will inevitably result in retarded healing. Removal of bacteria before adhesion occurs is a useful aid to wound healing. Antibiotics are used to treat known or suspected infections, and as prophylaxis for various types of medical and surgical procedures. Antibiotics seldom eliminate infection; rather they reduce the rate of bacterial replication to a degree, which allows the host's defence systems to eliminate the infectious agent.

The side-effects of antibiotics include:
1. Bacterial resistance.
2. Anaphylactic reactions.
3. Overgrowth of bacteria and gastrointestinal disturbances.
4. Specific toxicity on organs and systems.

Tetanus vaccination status should be established in all cases. If the horse has had a recent vaccination then there should be no risk of the disease, as the vaccine is highly effective. Where the vaccination history is dubious, either a tetanus toxoid booster vaccination or antiserum (or both) should be administered.

Protocol for Best Practice Use of Antibiotics (Figure 37)

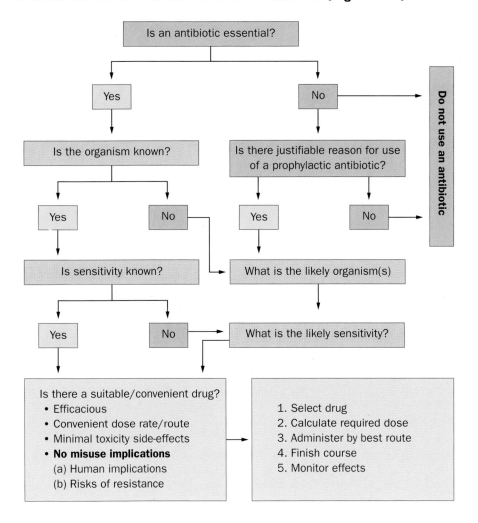

Wound Lavage

Wound lavage is an essential part of the management of fresh and older wounds. It is used to remove adherent and non-adherent bacteria and foreign matter from the wound without compromising the physiological status of the tissues involved. The two major factors are the type of fluid used and the pressure of the fluid used.

Given the essential need for a physiologically sound fluid, the pressure is more important than the actual fluid used; in order to overcome bacterial adhesion the ideal pressure is 10–15 psi (as achieved by commercially available lavage instruments such as a 'Water-Pic'. However, a 35/50 ml syringe with a 19G needle attached will provide about 8 psi.

The Mills wound irrigator is an ideal safe and convenient wound irrigation system. It can be attached to a bag of sterile saline without any difficulty or delays, so that the wound can be lavaged with an ideal solution at an ideal pressure.

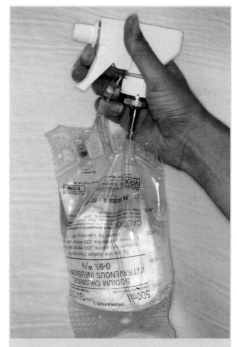

Figure 38 The Mills wound irrigator system provides physiologically sound, sterile irrigation at an ideal pressure. It is both convenient and efficient.

Lavage Fluids

Saline (Physiological Saline)

Saline is the ideal irrigation solution because of its physiological compatibility. It can be delivered from a sterile injection bag, but a working solution in large volumes can be made by adding a flat teaspoonful of salt to 0.6 liters (1 pint) of warm (previously boiled) water. Saline can be used to restore physiological normality after water irrigations have been used.

Water

Fresh clean (drinking) water is probably sterile enough as an initial wound lavage fluid, but it lacks physiological compatibility and has the potential to cause cell swelling. Prolonged and repeated water irrigation can cause significant cell destruction. It should not be used apart from initial 'washing of gross contamination' if saline is available, and in any case its use should be followed by saline to restore normal physiological status.

Povidone Iodine

Povidone iodine is commonly supplied as a 10% solution. The active ingredient is free iodine; dilute (0.1–1%) solutions have greater bactericidal activity than the full strength product. Serum can reduce activity (by binding free iodine) and there is only a short-lived residual effect, hence if used to maintain cleanliness of a wound, 4–6 hourly repetition is necessary.

Strong solutions of povidone iodine can be detrimental to healing, even causing necrosis; 0.1–0.5% solutions can be used for lavage purposes.

The benefit of povidone iodine in controlling bacterial infection may be limited. Povidone iodine solutions can cause nerve damage if they are repeatedly applied to exposed nerves.

Chlorhexidine

Chlorhexidine is a broadly active antiseptic. It is usually supplied in 10% solution in a soap base as a surgical scrub. When mixed with saline it forms a precipitate within only 12–24 hours. If solutions must be stored, deionized water should be used as the diluent. The advised concentration is 0.05% to avoid adverse effects on the tissues. Irrigation with 0.05%–1% chlorhexidine solutions probably leads to fewer infections when compared to 0.1%–0.5% povidone iodine. It also has a significant residual activity, being bound to cells.

Hydrogen Peroxide

Hydrogen peroxide is available in various strengths measured in volumes of oxygen released (the strongest solution is 30 volumes). Solutions over five volumes will cause tissue damage. While various solutions have been used for wound lavage, it is now generally considered unsuitable for this purpose because of the tissue damage it causes. Hydrogen peroxide can however, be used as a debriding agent and for flushing out anaerobic wounds (e.g. in the sole of the foot).

Acetic/Malic/Salicylic Acid

Commercial mixtures of these (and other) acids are available as wound irrigation solutions, but they are very acidic and highly tissue toxic. They are totally unsuitable as initial wound lavage solutions and should be reserved for special purposes only. Application of the solutions to a fresh wound results in the wound turning black due to formation of acid hematin. These solutions should be used only when *Pseudomonas* spp. infection is suspected or proven. Under these conditions they can be very effective.

The ointment forms can be useful debriding agents in the early stages of management of neglected, infected, and highly contaminated wounds.

Soluble Antibiotics

Dilute antibiotic solutions, e.g. penicillin, ampicillin, neomycin, kanamycin, and gentamicin, have been beneficial when added to lavage solutions. However, the solutions usually have an inappropriate pH for wound healing, and so some cell damage is expected. Suspensions of antibiotics and ointments are not appropriate for wound lavage. Antibiotic creams used for bovine mastitis treatment are not suitable for wound management and should never be applied to a healing wound.

Skin Wound Repair

Suture Patterns

Sutures are used to close a wound and are used for first intention (primary union) healing (Table 3). Sutures are also used in delayed primary healing. The decision to suture a wound must be based on sound understanding of the likely healing processes involved. Primary closure is the best method of closing and healing a skin wound, but is only applicable to a relatively narrow range of accidental wounds that fulfill certain criteria: the wound should be fresh, clean, and there should be no foreign matter within the wound bed. In addition, once closed by suturing there should be no tension on the wound (unless suitable tension relieving mechanisms can be applied), including during movement or swelling, and there should be no dead space within the wound.

Table 3 Suture materials for skin closure

Absorbable

Name	Material	Character	Gauges (metric)	T1/2 (days)	Color
Vicryl	Polyglactin 910	Synthetic braided-coated	0.4–8	14	Purple
Vicryl Rapide	Polyglactin	Synthetic braided-coated	0.6–5	7	Purple/white
Dexon	Polyglycolic acid	Synthetic braided	0.7–5	10	Green
PDS	Polydioxanone	Synthetic monofilament	0.5–5	35	Blue
Maxon	Polyglyconate	Synthetic braided-coated	0.4–8	14	Green

Non-absorbable

Name	Material	Character	Gauges (metric)	T1/2 (days)	Color
Supramid	Polyamide (nyl)	Synthetic sheathed	0.5–8	N/a	White
Vetafil	Polyamide	Synthetic sheathed	1.5–7	N/a	White
Ethibond	Polyester	Synthetic braided-coated	0.5–7	N/a	Green
Ethilon	Polyamide (nyl)	Synthetic monofilament	0.7–5	N/a	Blue
Prolene	Polypropylene	Synthetic monofilament	1–4	N/a	Blue
Mersilk	Silk	Natural braided	0.2–5	N/a	Black
	Linen	Natural braided	2–5	N/a	White
Michels clips	Stainless steel	Synthetic	–	N/a	Metal

Simple Interrupted Sutures (Figure 39)

Advantages: These are multiple sutures each taking its own proportion of the tension across the wound. If one is disrupted it does not affect the others. They are simple to insert and remove, and provide reasonable cosmesis.

Disadvantages: They are slow to close an extensive wound, and there can be difficulty with apposition of tissue. Overall tension relief is probably poor, with too much tension applied to the suture and the immediately adjacent skin.

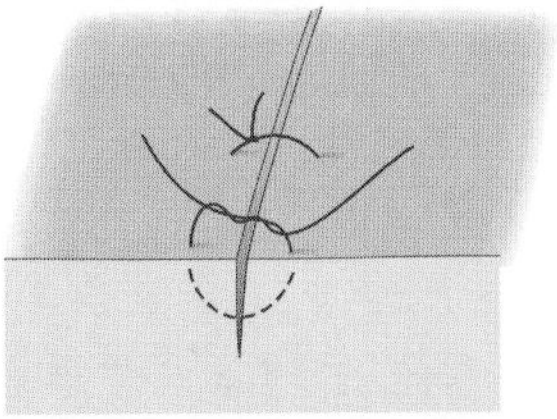

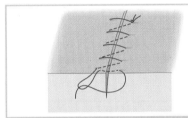

Figure 39 The suture is made by a single 'bite' through the tissue on each side and the knot is drawn away from the apposed wound margin.

Simple Continuous Sutures (Figure 40)

Advantages: This is a simple technique requiring no special skills. Tension in the suture is even throughout the length of the wound, and tension relief at the wound site is reasonable.

Disadvantages: If one part breaks down then the whole suture line is loosened by the appropriate amount. Removal can be slow if tension is not even. The wound is susceptible to larger amounts of foreign material due to potential gaps between the sutures. There is no special ability to appose the skin wound margins.

Figure 40 The initial simple suture is tied and one end is then carried forward to repeat the process to the end of the wound in slightly oblique parallel bites. The final knot is formed from the double end of the suture material and the loop of the last stitch.

Forward Overlocking (Continuous) (Blanket) Sutures (Figure 41)

Advantages: These provide rapid closure, with even tension along the length of the wound. The tension relief is effectively spread along the wound.

Disadvantages: The result is cosmetically poor, with a tendency to pucker skin at some point. Removal is slow.

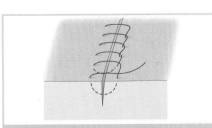

Figure 41 The suture is started as for the simple continuous suture but is continued as paralled bites with a return through the previous loop. The knot is ended as for the simple continuous suture.

Horizontal Mattress (Interrupted or Continuous) Sutures (Figure 42)

Advantages: With these sutures high tension relief can be maintained. They are strong and are unlikely to break down. The technique is simple and takes the knot away from the wound margin. No suture material is in contact with the actual wound edge.

Disadvantages: They are slow to insert and may cause necrosis of skin (and dehiscence) if under too much tension. The wound edges are not brought into apposition. The result is poor cosmesis with eversion of skin margins. Eversion means that extra skin is required and so it is not appropriate in every situation.

Vertical Mattress Sutures (Figure 43)

Advantages: These provide efficient tension relief with good apposition of wound margins. The result is cosmetically good.

Disadvantages: The sutures need careful placement, and more sutures are required. The technique uses double needle penetration on each side of the wound, so that the margins of the wound need to be healthy.

Subcuticular Sutures (Figure 44)

Advantages: Careful placement of these sutures is essential (especially of the knots at each end). They provide excellent cosmetic effects (sutures are invisible), with no opportunity for ingress of infection down the suture tracts.

Disadvantages: They are difficult to place when the skin is tightly fixed. Tension is difficult to equalize along the wound. Healing relies on complete resorption of suture material from the site (so it is essential to use absorbable suture material). Break down is potentially more likely and results in significant loss of tension along the whole suture line.

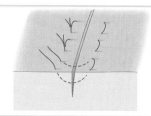

Figure 42 An initial deep bite is taken and then returned at the same depth. The knot lies below the two upturned wound margins.

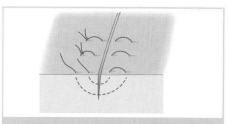

Figure 43 A deep bite is taken as for a simple interrupted suture and then very shallow 'return' bites are taken directly above the first deep bite to appose the skin margins.

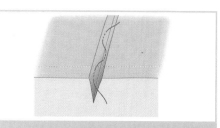

Figure 44 The first knot is placed subcutaneously and tied. Repeated horizontal bites are taken on opposite sides of the wound remaining in the subcuticular tissue. The last knot is tied deeply and the free end is drawn distally by inserting the needle through the skin the same distance away from the wound and cutting it off under mild tension.

Supported Quill Sutures (Figures 45, 46)

Advantages: These sutures provide extra tension relief of the wound margin, and are useful supportive sutures for other types in the wound itself. Distribution of tension can be varied according to the needs. Sutures can be tied in such a way as to enable release and retensioning as the wound heals.

Disadvantages: They are slow to insert and excessive tension is easy to obtain, which can cause dehiscence. Some necrosis is possible under the quills themselves.

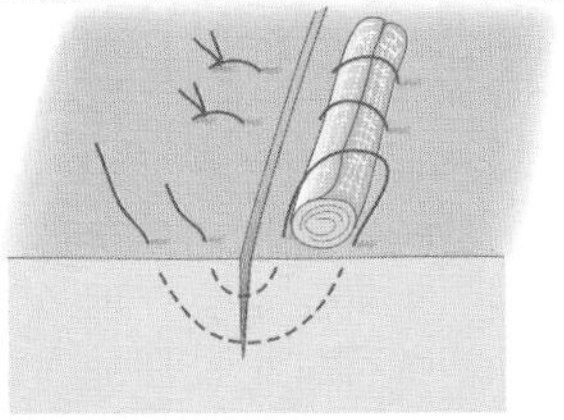

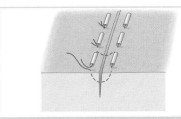

Figure 45 A vertical mattress suture is laid to include a stent on one or both sides of the wound margin

'Walking' Sutures

Advantages: These reduce dead space and maximize the possibility of reattachment of skin. The sutures minimize accumulation of fluid in the subcutaneous wound space, and reduce tension and minimize contraction of the skin. They provide close adhesion between skin and subcutis so that revascularization can take place.

Disadvantages: They are difficult and tedious to place enough to be helpful. One or two sutures alone are not very much use. Foreign material embedded in the wound may act as a nidus for infection.

Figure 46 A horizontal mattress suture is laid with short pieces of soft rubber or plastic tubing on either side of the suture. The tube should be the same length as the horizontal displacement of the suture to avoid distortion.

Staples (Figure 47)

Advantages: Staples can be rapidly inserted, and multiple staples can be used easily. They involve no skin penetration, so the margins of the wound are held in apposition with minimal skin trauma. The material is totally inert and has no foreign body implications.

Disadvantages: The major disadvantage is the lack of tissue volume held in each staple: the size is fixed and little adjustment is available. The skin needs to be positioned manually before the gun is fired to deliver a staple. Removal needs a special implement.

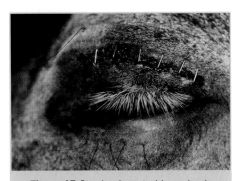

Figure 47 Staples inserted in a simple skin laceration in the upper eyelid.

Tissue Super-Adhesives

These are based around the long chain n-isobutyl cyanomethacrylate adhesives (SuperGlue). The adhesives require tissue moisture for full adhesion and this is maintained for 4–6 days. However, continuous soaking will eventually release the adhesion. The advantages of the modern tissue adhesives include the fact that they are less exothermic and have some flexibility. They are extremely powerful and adhesion is instantaneous. They have an added use in reinforcing other methods of closure (such as staples or sutures), and in supporting adhesive dressings in sites where a primary and secondary dressing cannot easily be retained.

Advantages: Adhesives provide rapid and powerful adhesion. They are convenient in small skin superficial lacerations, or where local anesthesia and sutures would either take too long or would preclude the horse from continuing the event. Adhesives have a hemostatic effect and little or no tissue toxicity. They result in a flexible wound site (using the new generation of adhesives; industrial superglues are not appropriate for tissue).

Disadvantages: They are only applicable to superficial incised wounds. Closure is temporary, continued tissue fluid contact will usually cause break down of adhesion within 2–5 days. The closure cannot easily be corrected if it is not precise when the glue is applied, and there are risks of contact between the injury and the surgeon's fingers! Cracking and breakdown is also a problem if the older types or domestic Superglue is used.

Stents (Figure 48)

Stents provide support for the margins of the wound and cover the wound site itself. They are very useful in horses where bandages cannot be applied, such as the body and head.

Advantages: Stents provide support for wound margins, and a covering for wound sites in locations that cannot be dressed with bandages. They maintain an even pressure on the wound site and so reduce fluid accumulation and dead space in the wound. Stents prevent bacterial contamination/infection at sites that cannot be covered by other means. A stent constructed from a non-felting swab soaked in hydrogel is an effective physiologically sound means of encouraging healing.

Disadvantages: Stents are time consuming to construct, and may cause tension on skin away from the wound which may not be ideal (especially on limbs), and extra skin trauma at the wound site. The covering over the wound is not usually replaceable unless tape sutures are used, and the wound site cannot be examined easily.

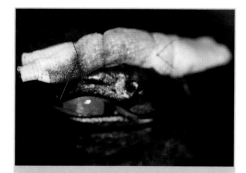

Figure 48 A stent constructed from a gauze swab soaked in hydrogel applied to an eyelid wound.

Drains (Figure 49)

Excess fluids and exudates can be harmful to wound healing because they can disrupt fascial planes, keep healing tissues apart, and harbor infection. Some wounds allow natural drainage of fluids by gravity, and this can be encouraged by suitable partial closure of a wound or by placing a surgical incision in such a way that drainage occurs (usually at the most dependent part of the wound). Drains are used to remove accumulated fluids from a closed or partially closed wound site.

The placement of the drain is critical to its function and it should not be simply laid through the wound under the skin because it will not function correctly; it may then act as a foreign body and hinder healing rather than helping it. Drains must be placed deep in the wound and should exit some distance from the end of the wound. Gravity must be used to assist the capillarity that is the main method of function. Drains are usually placed into or through a tissue plane that already has, or is expected to, accumulate fluid.

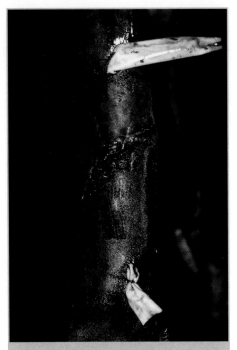

Figure 49 A Penrose drain inserted into the depths of a wound on the flexor aspect of a forelimb. Note the remote exit points.

Surgical drains are usually classified as active or passive. Active drains function mechanically (by suction or pressure), while passive drains rely on gravity or capillarity (or both). Simply creating or leaving a path for gravity seepage of fluid can instigate passive drainage from a wound site.

Drain Types

Drains reliant on capillary effects use rubber/latex or other materials. Tubular or flaccid (compliable) latex drains (e.g. Penrose drains) are in common usage in equine wound management. In the case of latex drains, there is no intraluminal drainage, all the fluid is lost by surface tension forces and, in fact, creating holes in the tubing reduces the effect. The drains are simple to use and remain effective until removed.

Bandage Drains (Seton)

These are used mainly to keep a draining sinus tract open. A length of cotton bandage is simply passed through the cavity of the wound and allowed to drain. The bandage can be moved back and forth to encourage drainage and delay healing until the wound is ready to close. This is a crude form of drain and the drain itself may allow infection to gain access to the wound site, or bits of bandage may separate and act as foreign bodies in the wound.

53

Tube Drains

Semi-rigid fenestrated tubular PVC or silastic drains work well provided that they do not become blocked with fibrinous exudates. They also provide a route for flushing of the wound. The fenestrated tube is laid deep within the wound, and is flushed from time to time to maintain its patency. These drains seldom work for long because the fenestrations rapidly become blocked by exudate and fibrin. They are most often used for draining the pleural and abdominal cavities.

When used for the chest, a one-way valve is placed on the open end to prevent aspiration of air. A suitable one-way valve is available commercially (Heimlich Valve), but a cheap and effective alterative is a finger of a polythene glove or a condom with the tip cut off and attached to the end of the tube. Fluid is actively expelled from the chest during expiration.

Active Vacuum (or Suction) Drains

These rely on a fenestrated tube and a persistent mild vacuum applied to the closed system that is left fastened to the open end of the drain (by a large syringe or purpose-made concertina pack system). Fluid is actively withdrawn from the wound site under persistent mild suction. Fluid is drawn into the canister so it is possible to obtain a good sense of how much exudate is being produced, and to obtain good material for culture and sensitivity from the depths of the wound without the complication of superficial skin infective organisms.

This is a common method used for chest and abdominal wounds where exudate enters and accumulates within the body cavities. Thoracic (pleural) or peritoneal drains are particularly useful in the management of open cavity wounds. Placement can be problematical, but modern one-way valve systems make them effective and relatively safe. Usually they are gravity fed, or in the case of thoracic drains, pressure fed. Typically they should be removed as soon as their function is achieved.

Advantages: Drains remove excessive fluids arising in the wound bed and so effectively reduce dead space. They also remove the products of necrosis and inflammation.

Disadvantages: Drains can cause foreign body effects: the drain itself may induce a significant volume of the fluid. They may act as a 'wick' for infection to gain access to the wound site, so regular bacteriological testing is required, and usually antibiotics are given at least until the drain is removed. Culture taken directly from the drain on removal is often helpful. Placement is not always easy, and usually requires a new drainage portal for egress of fluid. Drains must be removed at an appropriate time before any ascending infection can develop.

Bandages, Dressings and Dressing Techniques

Dressings are used to assist the management of wound sites, and allow the microclimate of the wound to be manipulated to the benefit of wound healing. Limb bandages must be applied with a full understanding of the local anatomy and should take account of the special requirements for the particular wound.

Some areas cannot easily be bandaged but a dressing can usually be fashioned that will at least provide some protection and support for the injured skin and other tissues. (See Figure 51 for upper limb and buttock bandages). All dressings and materials applied to wounds must be physiologically sound. Modern wound dressings such as hydrogels, calcium and sodium alginate, and absorptive primary or secondary dressings have made the concept of dressings more scientific. The healing of any wound is strongly dependent on the measures taken in the first few hours, and dressings play an important role in this stage of wound management. Owners can easily be instructed in simple bandaging techniques in anticipation of a later injury to their horse, or can be taught how to apply dressing changes between clinical examinations.

Older dressings (some are still widely used) relied upon various forms of cotton or gauze. Gamgee tissue and cotton wool have been used for many years and still have a place (albeit restricted) in modern wound management. Dressing technology is based around human wound management; there is little research on the specific needs of equine wounds and so the clinician will need to make careful clinical judgments on the state of the wound at each dressing change.

Aims of a Dressing

Historically dressings had a passive role in wound healing, being used simply to conceal and cover wounds. The concept of moist wound management[10] meant that dressings have become an active component of wound management. Modern medical practice recognizes that a moist environment allows enhanced migration of epithelial cells, precludes trauma at the wound site either while it is in place or on removal, reduces the pain at the site of the wound, and actively contributes to gaseous exchanges at the wound site.

Modern dressings play an active role in wound management, and selection of the most appropriate type will make a significant contribution to the healing of the wound. By the same token, selection of the wrong dressing may be harmful to wound healing. There is no single dressing that is suitable for all stages of all wounds; there are no wounds that will require a single dressing from injury to healing.

The primary objectives of a dressing are:
1. To enhance and support the healing process.
2. To decrease contamination and further infection at the wound site.
3. To minimize edema by applying even firm pressure to the local tissues.
4. To absorb exudate.
5. To maintain a high humidity at the wound–dressing interface and so maintain a moist wound environment.
6. To maintain local temperature and insulate the area against variations of ambient temperature.
7. To lower the pH at the site (by creating a slightly acid environment relative to normal tissues).
8. To allow gaseous exchange.
9. To immobilize the wound site and so negate the harmful effects of movement.
10. To protect the site from further trauma.

There are no dressings that fulfill all these criteria in all conditions. The ideal dressing should be free of toxic or particulate matter, be conveniently packed in a sterile fashion, and suitably shaped to allow easy placement without significant risk to the wound site or the surrounding tissues. In addition, dressings should be easily removed without undue trauma to the healing tissues, and economically feasible.

Dressings Changes

Modern wound dressings can be selected carefully to suit the particular wound situation. Thus, for an exudative wound a highly absorptive dressing can be applied, but if such a dressing (e.g. an alginate) is applied to a dry wound it may result in harmful desiccation.

Dressings are always expensive, and in any case over-frequent dressing changes can often be harmful. There are no hard and fast rules about changing of dressings, but they should probably not be changed unless there is a genuine clinical reason for doing so. Many can safely be left for up to 4–6 days, but where there are overt complications or there are risks of skin damage due to the dressing itself then changes can justifiably be done sooner rather than later.

It is important that dressing changes are made before exudate seeps through to the external layer of a bandage ('strike-through'), to prevent the 'wicking' of bacteria inwards to the wound, or any significant bacterial overgrowth occurs in the wound site. Changes should be made before there is any damage to the site, either from the bandage itself or the exudate, which may result in tissue necrosis and maceration respectively.

Wound Dressings

A large number of wound dressings are now available to the clinician, and it is impossible to describe them all. However, the main groups of dressings used in horses are described in this section with their major uses, advantages, and disadvantages. The technology is advancing very rapidly, and new materials are being developed almost daily. The over-riding philosophy must be that careful selection of the best and most appropriate dressing for the particular stage of healing for particular wounds will result in a more rapid and better repair with more rapid return to normal use.

Layers of a Bandage

A wound will usually be dressed with a topical antibiotic or other material and then a primary dressing. The primary dressing is maintained in place by a secondary dressing, and then various types of tertiary dressing suitable for the location and purpose will be applied.

Primary or Contact Layer

Adherent dressings such as gauze can aid in the early debridement of a wound, but otherwise are too traumatic at removal to be recommended. They should not therefore be used during the repair phase of wound healing. The historical 'wet-to-dry' technique in which a wet gauze swab was applied directly to the wound surface and removed after it had become dry and adherent to the wound surface is of very little (if any) value in wound management. There is limited value in using this as an initial debriding technique but it has no physiological rationale.

Non-adherent dressings do not cause significant damage on removal. Polymeric foam dressing absorbs exudate and cushions the wound. Petroleum jelly impregnated wide gauze dressings are open-weave fabrics impregnated with soft paraffin. These allow the passage of exudate to the absorptive layers above. In common use in veterinary practice is a perforated film absorbent dressing with a non-adherent surface consisting of cotton viscose and acrylic fiber bonded to a perforated polyester film that is placed directly onto the wound (Melolin; Smith and Nephew).

Dressings utilizing the 'moist wound healing principle' include hydrogels (e.g. Intra-site; Smith and Nephew), hydrocolloids, and calcium alginate dressing, which is a dressing with hemostatic properties and high absorbency used for exudative wounds. Alginate dressings should not be used on dry wounds because they desiccate the wound site.

Polysaccharide paste (Debrisan; Pharmacia Upjohn) consists of small porous beads that absorb water to form a soft gel-like mass, with molecules of molecular weight over 5000 remaining in the space in-between. In man it has been shown that bacteria are carried away from the wound with the greatest numbers located in the surface layer.

Thin, transparent sheets of polyurethane backed with adhesive (OpSite; Smith and Nephew) can be useful over donor sites for skin grafts and on minor abrasions in horses.

Primary Dressings Materials

These are materials that are applied directly to the wound site. In some cases they are adhesive, and include the materials that are used to maintain moist wound healing conditions.

Hydrogels

Hydrogels donate moisture to the wound while sustaining and enhancing a moist wound healing environment without maceration of the tissues. While there are many variations they all conform to the same basic principles. Some, however, are better at donating fluid to the wound, and some are better at preventing ingress of infection. They are all physiologically sound and will provide healthy protection for a healing wound.

Advantages: Hydrogels are physiologically sound and donate moisture to the wound site.

Disadvantages: They are expensive, require a primary dressing to maintain their relationship to the wound, and not all adhere readily to the wound site.

Hydrocolloids

These are composite products based on naturally occurring hydrophilic polymers. They usually consist of a pressure sensitive adhesive skin contact layer that provides good adhesion to shaven skin. The adhesive absorbs water from the skin (in the non-wound area), and so modifies the adhesive to maintain a progressively higher level of adhesion. The hydrocolloid absorbs exudate in the wound site and forms a gel. The dressings usually include a water- and vaporproof backing and so the wound site becomes, in effect, an environmental chamber that is strongly adhesed to the surrounding skin. The expanding gel is gently forced into the wound site.

Advantages: The adhesive nature means that the dressing is strongly fixed to the wound site and will not usually migrate. The wound site remains in a moist gel that is conducive to healing. Frequent dressings changes are not necessary.

Disadvantages: Hydrocolloids are expensive, and the adhesive is not as good on haired skin (clipping is required). They are not easily removed, and are inclined to cause skin and wound surface trauma. It is difficult to know what is going on at the wound site under such a dressing.

Collagen Dressings

Collagen dressings are usually based on bovine type 1 collagen (Collplast; Naturin, UK). They are applied directly to the wound, and the premise is that this will provide a suitable and hospitable environment for migration of cells; thus short-circuiting the development of endogenous collagen. The dressings are either available as an adhesive plaster based dry dressing (that relies on wound fluid to activate the collagen), or as a powder form of collagen. The adhesives used in the commercial forms are excellent and it is possible to stick a plaster over a relatively small wound on clipped skin and it will usually remain *in situ* for several days.

Advantages: These dressings are relatively cheap, are a small convenient size, and have a strong adhesive. They are physiologically sound.

Disadvantages: Only small sizes are available so these dressings are only applicable to small wounds. They have initial desiccation effects, and the collagen type may not be conducive to cell migration in equine wounds.

Alginates

Alginates are derived mainly from certain species of seaweed. The alginates are produced commercially in flat-layered fabric type dressings, or in fleece or rope format. When applied to a bleeding surface the fibrous nature of the dressing and the high calcium ion content contribute to coagulation. Absorption of serum results in gel formation. The dressings are net abstractors of fluid from the wound site, and are therefore useful in bleeding wounds and in wounds with high exudate.

Advantages: Alginates are hemostatic, absorptive, and are easily removed at dressing change with minimal local trauma.

Disadvantages: Alginates are net abstractors of fluid; if applied to a dry or semi-dry wound, they are inclined to desiccate the wound site. They are also expensive, and are non-adhesive so are inclined to migrate away from the wound site.

Permeable sheets

These are commonly used as primary dressings in horses. They are available in sheets of various sizes and some have a waterproof backing. In exudative wounds a further absorptive dressing can be used over this.

Advantages: Sheets are cheap and very easy to use, and are non-adherent and so are easily removed at dressing changes. Permeable sheets maintain a reasonable moist wound healing surface.

Disadvantages: They have a very limited absorptive capacity, and are inclined to migrate away from the wound (unless an adhesive form is used).

Activated Charcoal

Activated charcoal dressings are used to control odor and absorb bacteria and some other wound debris. Additionally, they may have an inhibitory effect on granulation tissue.

Advantages: Activated charcoal dressings are readily available in a variety of sizes, have a strong deodorant effect, and absorb bacteria away from the wound surface. They are non-adherent, and are relatively cheap. The dressings have an inhibitive effect on granulation tissue, and the net construction delays 'strike-through'.

Disadvantages: A limited volume of exudate can be absorbed by these dressings, which do not contribute moisture to the wound site. They are only available in non-adhesive forms, so tend to migrate away from the wound site.

Hydrophilic Polymeric (Polyurethane) Foams

Polyurethane foam dressings are available as sheets and are usually backed by a waterproof but gas permeable backing sheet. They are designed to absorb exudate whilst still maintaining a moist wound surface. They may be adhesive and where this is the case the adhesive is non-effective on moist surfaces, and so the dressing does not adhere to the wound surface itself. Some have excellent adhesion to haired skin. They have an absorptive material held behind a one-way moisture membrane; fluid is absorbed from the wound site into the foam center. They are readily conformable and have been constructed into various shapes suitable for cavity wound management.

Advantages: They are easily managed in various sizes of sheet and shapes of cavity dressings. An almost ideal wound environment is maintained, and they are ideally suited to use with a hydrogel. The cushioned backing protects the wound site from trauma, and the dressing can be left *in situ* safely and no external wicking can occur. The adhesive forms do not migrate but the adhesive is not very strong (fluid negates its effects).

Disadvantages: Non-adhesive forms migrate away from the wound site and so retention is problematical.

Secondary Layer

The objective of the secondary layer is to provide support for the primary dressing, and also provide absorption and padding.

Soft synthetic orthopedic padding is frequently used (e.g. Soffban; Smith and Nephew) because it very soft and easy to handle. It cannot be over-tensioned because it simply tears. Non-elastic synthetic conforming bandages made from viscose, polyester, or cotton (or mixtures of these)) (e.g. Nephlex, Easifix; Smith and Nephew) provide a soft supportive first layer to retain the primary dressing in place. It is important that these are not pulled too tight.

Cotton wool can be easily molded around awkward areas. It is easy to unroll onto a limb rather like a giant thick, soft bandage, and is applied in the same standard fashion as a bandage. Simply removing the cotton wool over the site can relieve pressure areas such as the point of the hock and the accessory carpal bone (see p. 65).

Gamgee tissue (Robinson Animal Health, UK) is also used as a non-adherent primary/contact layer, and can be useful if it is cut to conform to the limb. It is very useful as a compact over-layer for cotton wool bases. However, it is very inclined to fold and does not conform well if it is used in its standard form as an initial secondary layer. It is, however, an effective component of a Robert Jones' bandage. A narrower width form is available that is more useful for standard dressings. A variety of cotton bandages are available for use in horses. They are classified as non-elastic or elastic, conforming or non-conforming. Disposable baby nappies are very effective in the early stages of the management of large wounds in absorbing the large amounts of exudate.

The width of the bandage is an important aspect of wound dressings. Narrow bandages tend to conform better than broader ones, but they also tend to put too much focal pressure onto the skin. Usually a 7–10 cm width is used in horses. The elasticized forms allow some conforming to occur, and tension can be spread through the dressing provided that the full elasticity is not used when applying the bandage.

Tertiary Layer

This secures and protects the primary/secondary layers, and may also have a supportive role. Adherent materials, (e.g. Elastoplast; Smith and Nephew) are adhesive and porous, but have minimal elasticity and therefore limited conforming ability. Because they stick to hair, they can be useful in preventing a dressing slipping down the limb. They are very strong and so it is easy to apply excessive tension when using these.

Self-adherent bandages stick only to themselves. They are typically elastic and hence conform well (e.g. Tensoplus Lite; Smith and Nephew). Dressings such as Coform Plus (Smith and Nephew) and Vetrap (3M) will not loosen with time or movement, and thus maintain constant pressure.

Non-adherent bandages may be disposable, e.g. crepe bandages, or re-usable, such as so-called 'exercise' (stretchy) or 'stable' (non-stretchy) bandages. Exercise bandages may shrink when dampened and this can lead to a compromise in blood supply if a bandaged limb or tail becomes wet.

Soft Cotton Bandage (Soffban)

This is a very soft (easily torn) bandage that is commonly used as secondary dressing (i.e. to retain the primary dressing). Rolls are rather short and so several may be required.

Cotton Bandages

Elasticized cotton bandages with conforming ability have considerable advantages over the non-elastic forms. The non-elastic forms provide good firm support, and can be used to provide greater pressure to the wound site. However, prolonged high pressure to the skin (especially of the limbs) must be avoided.

Pressage bandage

The pressage bandage is a reusable elasticized stocking with a zip fastener. It is available in different sizes for the tarsus (hock) region and the carpus (knee). It provides even pressure over the primary and secondary dressings, and can be applied as a secondary dressing in some circumstances when exudate is not a significant problem.

Application of a Dressing

Until the wound has granulated, any dressing applied serves two major functions, to absorb exudate and to prevent further trauma, contamination, and infection. In addition to the materials used, consideration should be given to how tightly the bandage should be applied; it should apply minimal pressure to avoid further compromise to the blood supply at the wound site. Once granulation tissue has filled any tissue deficit up to skin level, a firm pressure bandage will help to prevent it from becoming exuberant. Care should always be taken to avoid causing skin necrosis.

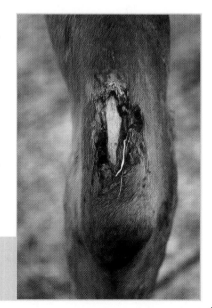

The most vulnerable sites are over the caudal edge of the accessory carpal bone in the forelimb, and over the Achilles tendon 5–10 cm above the point of the hock (Figure 50). Dressings that completely enclose the hock and the knee in particular, significantly restrict movement. Horses may resent restrictive movement (especially of the hock), and will often lift, abduct, and flex the hock quite vigorously. This maneuver may well partially disrupt the dressing, resulting in the point of the hock being exposed.

Figure 50 Skin and tendon necrosis arising from an overtight bandage (applied to treat a wound on the dorsal hock region).

A 'donut' of orthopedic felt or some other padding placed over the accessory bone will minimize the risk of a pressure sore. The Achilles region is best protected by placing a wad of padding on either side of the tendon to increase the area of contact. The point of the hock may be completely enclosed in the dressing or may be left uncovered. Either method is satisfactory (see p. 47).

The problem of bandages slipping down a leg can be overcome in several ways. These include using an adherent tertiary layer to stick the dressing to the limb, using a stretchy tertiary layer which will 'grip' better, and bandaging below the wound site before applying the dressing, to widen the diameter of the leg and hopefully prevent downwards movement.

The Head

Wounds on the head are particularly difficult to bandage; the nostrils, eyes, and mouth must be kept functional, and the jaws must be able to move freely without disturbing the bandage. The problems can be overcome partially by using adherent dressings (primary and tertiary).

Ocular and periocular wounds can be protected by placing a donut bandage over the area so that at least no further trauma can occur (Figure 83). Wounds around the eye and face can be dressed by using bandage stents, preferably impregnated with hydrogel, that are sutured over the site (Figure 48). These provide both protection and support for the wound site whilst maintaining a moist wound healing environment.

The Body Trunk (Figure 51)

Wounds on the body trunk are particularly difficult to dress but there are methods that can be useful albeit with limited cover. Bellybands and stents (made from Intrasite Conformable; Smith and Nephew or Surgipads) are useful.

Adhesive dressings can be useful and can remain in place for up to 48 hours without difficulty in most cases. The dressings are highly adhesive and the adhesion can be enhanced by the use of tissue adhesives.

The Upper Limb Regions (Figure 51)

The upper regions of the hind limb are almost impossible to bandage. The sharp taper to the thigh means that dressings are impossible to keep up. However, there are helpful methods that can be used to retain a dressing on the upper limb region or even on other sites such as the buttock, such as suturing the dressing to the skin, or placing retaining straps in the dressing. Although these only provide a limited cover they can be useful.

Stents (fashioned from rolled cotton swabs/Surgipads or conformable dressings) are useful in providing both tissue support and a clean dressing over the site of the wound. Stents soaked in hydrogel are particularly useful because they will maintain a moist wound healing environment.

Smaller adhesive dressings can be helpful, but movement and loss of adhesive properties can result in bandage loss. Firm veterinary adhesive bandages are available (e.g. Allevyn Adhesive

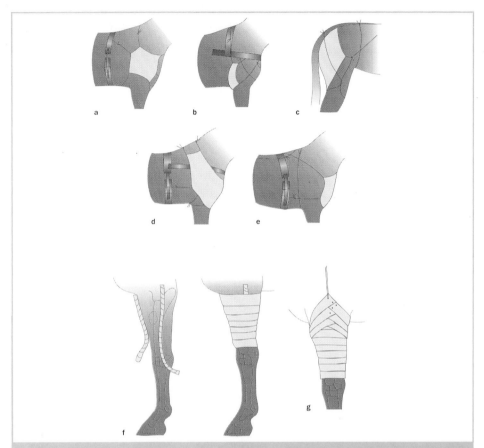

Figure 51 Bandaging upper limb regions. (a) Shoulder dressing; (b) elbow dressing; (c) buttock dressing; (d) breast and shoulder dressing; (e) breast dressing; (f) upper forelimb dressing showing a retention mechanism; (g) upper forelimb dressing retained by sutures and a support strap.

and Collplast collagen dressings), and the adhesive quality can be increased by the use of n-butyl cyanomethacrylate adhesives.

The Hock

The hock is a difficult site to bandage because of the range of movement and the resentment the horse feels when this is restricted. The major 'danger areas' are the common calcanean tendon (Achilles tendon) region (Figure 50), and the dorsal aspect of the hock below the tarsometatarsal joint. The point of the hock is also a potential danger point because of the thin skin cover and prominent bone of the tuber calices.

Dressings applied to the hock rely on the Achilles (common calcanean) tendon to keep them up. There are serious risks if the bandage is placed too tight and if it is too loose it will just fall off!

A loose bandage can move downwards and 'hang' on the Achilles tendon causing pressure damage (Figure 50). The problems can be overcome by careful placement of the pressure components of the dressings (the tertiary layers) (Figure 52).

Wounds on the point of the hock are particularly difficult to dress. A suitable shaped dressing is a useful aid. Dressing made specifically for the human heel (e.g. Allevyn Heel; Smith and Nephew) can be modified for horses, and provide an excellent method of applying a conforming primary dressing to these wounds. The seam may need to be relieved slightly for an ideal fit. This dressing will usually remain *in situ* so long as the secondary dressing is fully supportive.

With hock bandages applied to protect and support dorsal hock wounds there is a risk that the primary dressing will migrate out of the wound site. This can be avoided by using an adhesive primary dressing.

Movement is a serious difficulty. Many horses will resent any restriction to hock movement. After the dressing is applied many horses will flex the hock strongly and repeatedly. During forced flexion there is a high pressure on the Achilles tendon and the plantar region of the tarsus. During forced extension the forces are transferred to the dorsal aspect of the hock (Figure 52). If this occurs, the dressing must be checked again for tension over the calcanean tendon region, and if necessary replaced in its entirety.

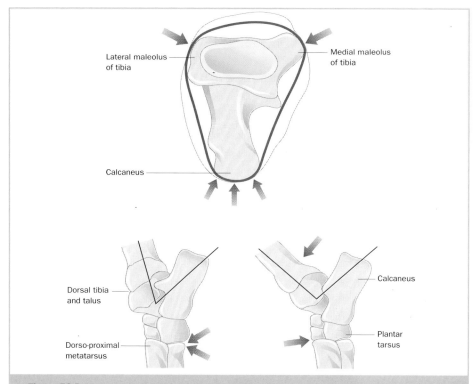

Figure 52 Pressure points at the level of the hock.

The risks can be minimized by ensuring that the point of the hock is protected by a purpose-made soft pad, or a plug of cotton wool can be removed from the site during the early stages of the cotton wool layers. A sympathetic figure-of-eight bandaging technique is used so that there is no tension on the Achilles tendon (a finger should be able to run over the tendon under the bandage at each stage. Including a roll of 10 cm wide cotton bandage (unopened) on either side in the hollow below the Achilles tendon after the primary and secondary dressings have been applied can be helpful. This will transfer the tension to the bandage roll. If the bandages are left sealed, they can be used at the next dressings change! Regular checks on the comfort and stability of the dressing should be made; if any dressing is obviously uncomfortable then it should be removed and replaced. Bandaging the hock is shown in Figure 53.

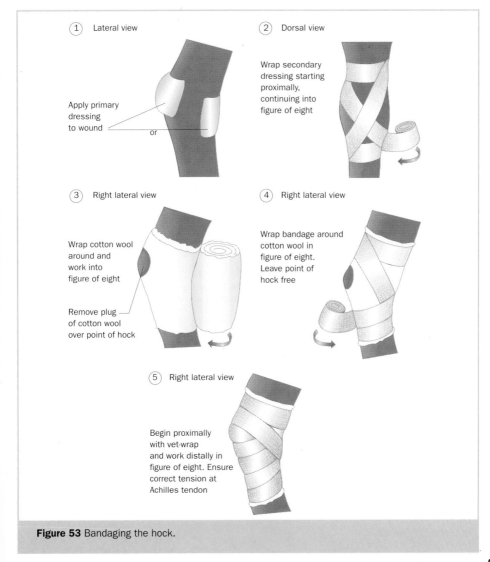

1 Lateral view

Apply primary dressing to wound

or

2 Dorsal view

Wrap secondary dressing starting proximally, continuing into figure of eight

3 Right lateral view

Wrap cotton wool around and work into figure of eight

Remove plug of cotton wool over point of hock

4 Right lateral view

Wrap bandage around cotton wool in figure of eight. Leave point of hock free

5 Right lateral view

Begin proximally with vet-wrap and work distally in figure of eight. Ensure correct tension at Achilles tendon

Figure 53 Bandaging the hock.

Bandaging the Knee

The knee is difficult to bandage because of the downwards taper of the area, although the knee itself is wider than the radius and the metacarpus.

The knee is a high motion joint, but fortunately horses tolerate immobilization of this area rather better than the hock.

The skin over the palmar aspect is particularly thin and the skin covering the accessory carpal bone comes under considerable pressure during flexion and extension of the carpus. The skin over the medial and lateral radial tuberosities is also thin and very closely related to the bone; it is very liable to pressure damage from bandages (Figure 54).

The problems can be addressed by ensuring that the accessory carpal bone area is left out of the first secondary layer, and by removing a plug of cotton wool from the first layer of cotton wool (Figure 55). A standard figure-of-eight bandage will usually stay in position well if applied properly. It is useful to use adhesive primary dressings for injuries on the dorsal aspect of the carpus. This will reduce the tendency for primary dressing slippage.

The dressing is applied using in a strong figure-of-eight format (Figure 55): after the primary dressing has been applied to the wound site it is retained by a secondary dressing of a soft cotton wool bandage applied in a figure-of-eight pattern. It is common practice at this stage to avoid covering the accessory carpal bone.

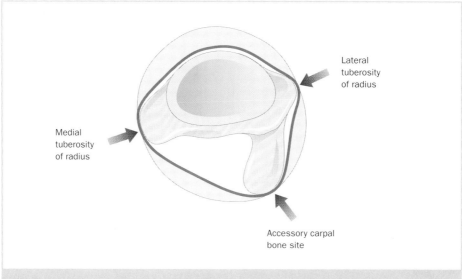

Lateral tuberosity of radius

Medial tuberosity of radius

Accessory carpal bone site

Figure 54 Pressure points at the level of the carpus.

A layer of cotton wool is placed over the secondary dressing in the same format (but covering the accessory carpal bone), and a plug of cotton wool is removed from over the bony prominence. A mildly elasticized cotton bandage is now applied in the same figure-of-eight, avoiding the accessory carpal region. The next layer of cotton wool is applied in a simple overlapping way to cover the whole area, and a cotton bandage and an elasticized adhesive layer cover this finally. In order to avoid slippage, it may be helpful to apply a bandage to the lower limb region first and then dress the carpus. A properly applied carpal bandage will probably not slip provided that the horse is box-rested.

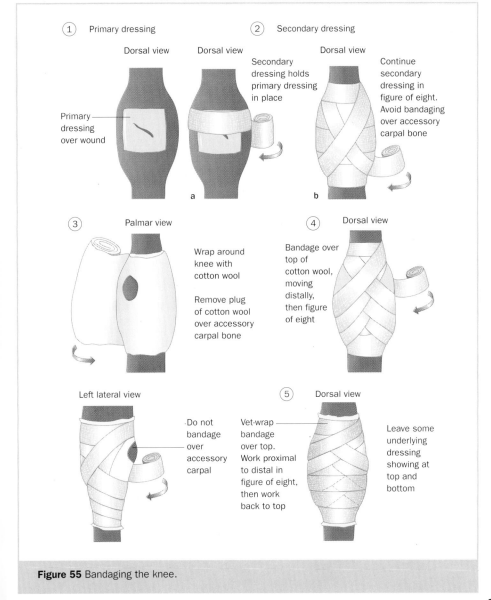

Figure 55 Bandaging the knee.

67

Bandaging the Fetlock

The fetlock region is relatively easy to bandage, and most owners are experienced in application of exercise bandages. However, pressure points over the palmar aspect of the fetlock (sesamoid region) can cause pressure wounds. A suitable protective pad can be placed over the region provided that there is no risk of it kinking and becoming a more serious problem itself. The bandage might ride up from the coronet and down from the metacarpus, creating a tight compressed band around the pastern or distal metacarpal/fetlock region. This can be very dangerous if the wound is exudative and if the tertiary layer is a non-elastic adhesive bandage.

Movement is difficult to reduce with a simple fetlock dressing. A Robert Jones' bandage (see p. 70) should be considered if movement is likely to be an important aspect of healing.

A suitable primary dressing should be applied and retained with a layer of cotton wool bandage using a figure-of-eight method, crossing over at the front of the fetlock and leaving the palmar area over the proximal sesamoids uncovered. A thin layer of cotton wool is then applied in normal spiral fashion overlapping each layer by 50%, followed by a simple cotton bandage (e.g. Nephlex, Smith and Nephew) in a similar fashion. A second layer of cotton wool should then be applied, and retained by a tertiary bandage of elasticized or adhesive dressing.

Bandaging the Foot (Figure 56)

The hoof is difficult to bandage because of the tendency for dressings to ride upwards onto the pastern, and because of the high 'wear-rate' of ambulatory patients.

The problem of 'riding upwards' can be minimized by ensuring that the bandage is extended downwards over the heels, and taking at least several layers under the heels of the hoof. A figure-of-eight bandage is effective.

The tendency to wear through after a short distance can be overcome by providing firm support with 'duck tape' type nylon reinforced tape. This should be applied around the solar margin of the hoof and extended onto the heels (but not onto the skin). Several layers may be needed, and it may be helpful to protect the sole with a multi-layer pad of 'duck tape', which is then folded up onto the walls before placing the encircling tape support. In any case this dressing must be checked regularly and reinforced if needed. The problem is worse if the foot is shod.

Bandages on the foot have a high tendency to become soaked with water, soiled bedding, or urine and feces. This means that wicking effects for infection are likely under most circumstances. In some cases the dressing can be protected from wet by placing the dressed foot into a high-density polythene bag and taping the bag onto the foot. It may be possible therefore to make the dressings waterproof but this may encourage sweating and heat and so this can be viewed as a disadvantage.

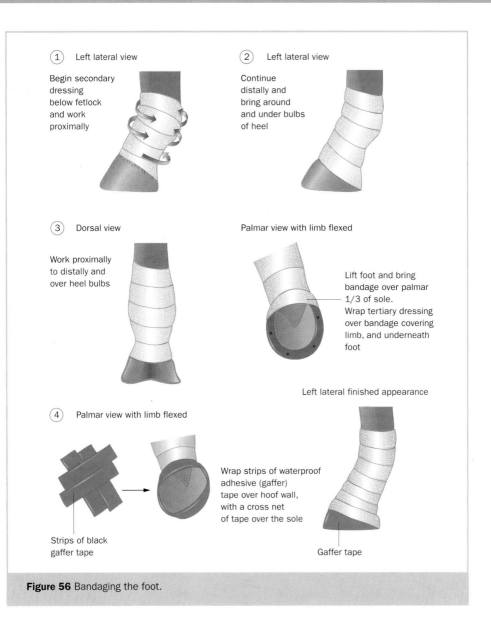

Figure 56 Bandaging the foot.

The Robert Jones' Bandage

This method of bandaging was developed to produce temporary immobilization of human limbs, and has several indications in equine practice. It can provide first aid support for a fractured limb or disrupted suspensory apparatus giving stability and soft tissue protection, and can be used to control severe post-trauma limb edema by application of even pressure. In addition it can be used to support a limb following removal of a more rigid external or internal fixation device, and to protect implants and soft tissues during recovery from anesthesia.

Note

The unreinforced Robert Jones' Bandage does not, on its own, completely restrict movement. Even when correctly applied some movement of the limb is possible.

In the event that movement is to be totally restricted the bandage must be supported with splints or an alternative method should be used.

The principle of the dressing is compression of air-filled cotton wool to increase rigidity and spread pressure evenly over the whole limb region included. To achieve this, the Robert Jones' bandage has to be multi-layered and bulky. The primary and secondary layers are applied as already described. Each layer of cotton wool approximately 2.5 cm thick is kept firmly in place with a gauze bandage, each layer being wrapped more tightly than the preceding one. The top two layers are usually pulled as tight as possible. Layers are applied until a total diameter of approximately three times that of the normal leg is achieved (20–25 cm for an adult, 15–20 cm for a foal). Additional rigidity can be achieved by incorporating rigid splints on the outer layers of the bandage, e.g. plastic guttering, broom handles, or wooden boards. A minimum of two splints should be used at 90° for optimum stability.

The completed bandage should be very firm and should respond like wood to a firm flick with the finger. It should prevent all movement of the limb and should provide useful support. The bandage may extend up to the carpus or hock, or may be full length and extend up to the elbow or stifle.

A full-length Robert Jones' bandage for a forelimb will require:
1. 10–12 x 500 g rolls of absorbent cotton wool.
2. 20–25 gauze bandages.
3. 4–6 rolls of non-elastic adhesive tape.

The primary dressing is retained by a suitable secondary dressing of soft cotton wool bandage and cotton wool is rolled onto the leg to give two layers over the entire length to be incorporated. A conforming cotton bandage is then drawn firmly over the entire length, avoiding pressure points. A further layer of cotton wool is placed over the entire length of the area concerned. Further bandages are then applied over the entire length (including pressure points). Successive layers of cotton wool and bandage are used to provide at least 4–6 layers. The top layer is secured with an adhesive non-elastic tape or broad nylon tape (carpet tape is effective and strong). Tape must never be used on the lower layers.

Precautions and Complications of Robert Jones' Bandages

The Robert Jones' bandage should be firm enough to prevent significant movement of the limb. However, it is probably not possible with an unsupported Robert Jones' bandage to restrict movement completely.

Failure to apply enough pressure may permit some movement, and this can result in serious creasing and pressure lines in the bottom layers.

Skin damage can occur, such as serious excoriation or scalding from exudative wounds. The bottom of the bandage is usually in contact with the ground and so 'wicking up' from wet/soiled bedding can be a problem. Movement restriction can be resented (particularly for hind limbs).

Rigid Limb Casting

Rigid limb casting can be a very significant aid to management of limb wounds in particular. Application of a cast is a specialized wound dressing technique that needs to be meticulously performed if problems are to be avoided. The advantages of casting should be balanced with the potential disadvantages.

Advantages: Apart from the obvious use of rigid limb casting in the management of orthopedic disorders such as fractures, rigid limb casting is a useful measure in the management of distal limb wounds, and in particular wounds of the hoof capsule, heel bulbs, and tendons. It is also a useful way of controlling movement during healing of limb lacerations involving the cannon, fetlock, and pastern region. The healing of bone, tendon, and ligament injuries (whether accompanied by skin wounds or not) can also be aided by casting. Not only is restriction of movement important, but also the restriction of space appears to be a factor in allowing wounds to heal without formation of exuberant granulation tissue.

Disadvantages: The wound cannot be assessed as simply as with changing bandages, and problems both with the wound site and the cast itself may only show when there is already a serious problem. Infection cannot easily be controlled or monitored, and exudate cannot be removed.

Casts can be removed without general anesthesia, but application is much more difficult. Once on, the cast has to remain as applied unless there are complications when a replacement strategy needs to be planned. Casts are expensive, although modern light and strong casting materials make the procedure more tolerable for the horse. Casting a limb may cause disuse osteopenia and tendon slackness. There may be complications to the other leg (including weight-bearing laminitis and tendon laxity/disruption) if the cast is not tolerated well.

Types of Cast

Foot only. This is most often used in the management of hoof capsule injuries and for restriction of movement in cases of pedal bone fracture. The casts are well tolerated and are very safe with minimal risks.

Half limb. This is the commonest form of rigid limb casting and is used on the limb up to the proximal cannon. It is easy to manage and monitor from day to day, and is usually well tolerated.

Full limb (Figure 57). These are very difficult to manage and are often poorly tolerated (especially for hind limbs). They are used for the proximal radius/tibia.

Tube cast. These are constructed from plastic guttering or piping and are used in foals for proximal fetlock to proximal radius/tibia injuries.

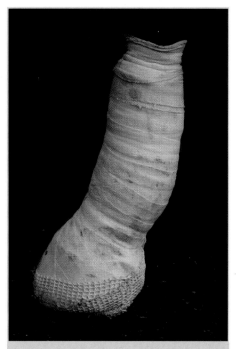

Figure 57 Half limb cast.

Specific wound or injury related indications for rigid limb casting include management of severe distal limb lacerations and partial hoof avulsions, support for injured soft tissues, e.g. tendon or ligament strains, and fracture fixation (sole or support for internal fixation). In addition, rigid limb casts can be useful in joint luxation/ligament injury (in unstable joint/ruptured ligament cases), and for the correction of developmental or acquired limb deformities. Emergency immobilization of the injured limb can be achieved by the use of a Monkey splint or other temporary fixation method (e.g. Farley boot).

Management of Horse with a Cast

Horses with a limb in a cast require careful monitoring to ensure that minor problems do not develop into serious ones. The horse must be confined to a loosebox, but should be walked out a few paces each day so that weight bearing can be monitored. The top of the cast must be protected from ingress of hay/shavings/water and so on, by using an adhesive tape collar. Twice daily checks on the cast are obligatory (walk a few paces, temperature [hot/cold], smell, exudate, swelling at proximal end, evidence of pain/dullness).

Casts applied as an aid to wound management seldom need to be on for more than 2–3 weeks and often immobilization for 1–2 weeks gives enough response. In general, casts should be removed as soon as they have had the desired effect. Comfortable foot and half limb casts are usually tolerated very well, but full limb casts are much more difficult.

Complications

Complications include pressure sores, cast movement or fracture/instability, and vascular obstruction (causing gangrene).

Weight-bearing laminitis or tendon disruption in the contralateral leg can also occur (usually from non-weight-bearing on the cast leg).

Signs of problems include increased reluctance to use the limb, a febrile response by the horse, or dullness and a tendency to lie down. Biting and chewing at the cast, excessive heat or profound cold of the cast, exudate seeping through at the site of the wound or at pressure points, and a fetid smell particularly at the top of the cast are all signs of problems. Swelling of the leg above the cast is a cause for alarm and warrants immediate renewal if the cast has not been used for an extensive soft tissue injury, when some swelling may be expected. These signs must not be ignored.

Often by the time the horse shows significant resentment or pain, serious skin (or deeper) necrosis may have occurred. This will be difficult to protect from further damage when the cast is replaced. Analgesics such as non-steroidal anti-inflammatory drugs may mask a serious problem, so doses should be used carefully and extra vigilance taken to monitor the cast. Loosening of the cast due to a combination of disuse muscle atrophy and reduction in swelling is more likely when large full length casts have been used.

Disuse osteopenia may occur particularly in young growing animals, and is most likely to affect the proximal sesamoid bones and phalanges. The process is reversed when the cast is removed and the patient starts to use the leg again. Pressure sores, or more commonly rubs, can occur despite meticulous application of a cast. Rubs most frequently occur over the abaxial surface of the proximal sesamoids, the proximal dorsal metacarpus (metatarsus), and the accessory carpal bone. Most will resolve merely by applying another cast provided this is not delayed.

Removal of Cast

A cast must not be placed unless there is a definite plan for its removal. Removal may be required within a very short time, and as soon as there are indications that suggest the cast is not safe and comfortable it must be removed immediately.

In the absence of complications, in adult horses a cast can be left in place for 3–4 weeks. This is usually long enough for almost all skin wounds to heal satisfactorily. In some cases however, the cast will need to be removed and replaced. Casts used to immobilize extensive soft tissue injury may require changing every 10–14 days, depending on the amount of wound drainage and suppuration. There are therefore two strategies that need to be considered: removal with replacement, and removal without replacement.

In the former case a general anesthetic may be indicated, while in the latter the cast may be removed simply under sedation. In foals, casts should be changed at least every 14 days because of limb growth within the cast. An oscillating plaster saw is essential to remove the cast. Cast saws are noisy and it is advisable to sedate the horse; anesthesia may be indicated in some cases both for management and medical reasons. Plugging the horse's ears with cotton wool sometimes helps. The cast should first be scored with the saw and then cut to full depth in small bites. Cuts are made on the medial and lateral sides of the leg and need to go through the whole thickness of the cast. Care must be taken not to cut the underlying skin.

The cast should not be removed until it can definitely be removed in one move (especially if the horse is conscious). The wire guide method for removal of a cast should not be used, except perhaps for the foot cast. Wire saw cuts could cause horrendous injuries unless the placement of the tubes at the time of casting is extremely accurate.

Summary

Applied correctly materials currently available can be relied upon not to break and provide a convenient means of providing strong, durable, external support to injured limbs. Cast failures regardless of the material used are costly and potentially very serious. At best they entail re-anesthetizing the horse and applying a stronger cast, at worst they can cause irreparable damage.

Management of Wound Exudate

Excessive wound exudate is unusual in horses. Extensive skin loss, burns, or large bleeding/granulomatous wound sites usually have the most exudate.

Exudate from a wound can be:
1. Hemorrhage (either capillary seeping or overt venous or arterial hemorrhage).
2. Serum/plasma exudation.
3. Inflammatory fluids (frequently infected).

The consequences of continued seepage of blood or plasma include protein loss, anemia (caused by direct blood loss or a chronic inflammatory process), and electrolyte and trace element (zinc, iron) loss.

Chronic protein loss needs to be matched by increased intake, and so unless the diet of the horse is adjusted clinically significant hypoproteinemia can arise. It is unlikely that the extent will be extreme, but even small reductions may adversely affect the general health of the patient.

Wounds that are characterized by wound exudate include burns, extensive grazing injuries, non-healing wounds with exuberant granulation tissue, and chronically infected, non-healing wounds. Exudate is also produced by large fibroblastic sarcoid lesions developing at wound sites, wounds involving large serous surfaces such as the peritoneum and pleurae, and wounds involving body ducts, secretory glands, and synovial membranes (e.g. salivary glands and ducts and joints).

Management of Exudate

The exudate should be controlled by appropriate wound management through:
1. The use of pressure bandages.
2. Placement of a suitable drain (Figure 49).
3. Surgical removal of infected or exuberant granulation tissue.
4. Treatment of fibroblastic sarcoid.
5. Restoration of synovial integrity or duct continuity.
6. Obliteration of secretory glands by surgical or chemical (or other) extirpation.

A healthy wound site consistent with normal healing should be maintained. Exudate results in improved opportunities for bacterial infection (which in turn increases the inflammatory response and so increases the amount of exudate), and results in tissue maceration. There is a significant difference between a moist wound healing environment and a macerated wound. The former will have an improved chance of healing while the latter will almost certainly fail to heal. Burns are notoriously exudative and must be managed particularly carefully.

The metabolic deficits should be restored through good nutrition and limitation of the losses. Blood and in particular protein status should be monitored regularly, and a healthy diet with trace element supplementation ensured.

Management of Granulation Tissue

Granulation tissue forms faster in horses than in ponies and this can result in the apparent (or actual) expansion of the wound site (Figure 58). Exuberant granulation tissue associated with refractory chronic inflammatory processes is a common complication of limb wounds of larger horses[12]. Many (if not all) accidental wounds naturally produce granulation tissue – indeed it is essential in most cases where repair is reliant on second intention or delayed primary union healing.

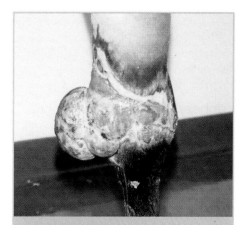

Figure 58 This wound had failed to heal for some months and the wound site had become much larger. Granulation tissue was exuberant.

In spite of the high incidence of exuberant granulation (proud flesh) in distal limb wounds of horses (as opposed to ponies), some distal limb wounds heal remarkably well with evidence of contraction and limited granulation. When excessive granulation tissue develops on wounds on the head or body trunk there is usually some definable reason, e.g. foreign body or necrotic tissue (see p. 28 and Figure 59).

The rate of production of granulation tissue can be *partially* controlled in some cases by limiting the extent of the inflammatory response through control of infection, removal of foreign bodies, and careful management of the early stages of the wound. Local (topical) corticosteroid therapy can be helpful, as can application of a pressure bandage or rigid limb cast. Restriction of movement by confining the horse to a loosebox, or application of firm bandages or even rigid limb casts is also useful.

Management

The nature of granulation tissue needs to be established. A significant number of cases involve either botriomycosis (staphylococcal pyogranuloma/bacterial pseudomycetoma) (see p. 27), or sarcoid transformation (see p. 31). Biopsy of a small representative portion of the tissue may be helpful, but in any case all tissue excised from wounds should be examined by a pathologist. In the event that the wound is complicated by pyogranuloma or sarcoid, healing cannot be expected unless all the affected tissue is removed.

Sarcoid affected granulation tissue is much more difficult to manage than pure granulation tissue or pyogranuloma (Figures 29, 34). Treatment must eliminate every single sarcoid cell, otherwise healing will not take place. However, there are currently no effective methods of categorical elimination of sarcoid cells from the site of wounds. Management of fibroblastic sarcoids on the distal limbs is particularly difficult, and the complications have been described[13].

Once sarcoid and staphylococcal pyogranuloma can be eliminated then other reasons for non-healing (see p. 25) should be eliminated. Even in complicated wounds, careful assessment and early management will likely result in some cases healing normally. Where all identifiable factors have been eliminated, idiopathic exuberant granulation tissue can be diagnosed and this can then be managed accordingly (see below).

Exuberant Granulation Tissue

Exuberant granulation tissue is best excised surgically, although application of corticosteroid based water-soluble creams may have a considerable effect on the depth and rate of proliferation of the tissue. Surgical excision may be required on a number of occasions before epithelium completely covers the wound (Figures 60, 61).

The absence of sensory nerves in granulation tissue usually means excision can be done in the standing horse without recourse to anesthesia. However, general anesthesia is often the best way to ensure complete and effective removal of all unhealthy tissue, particularly in long-standing or extensive wounds. The bed of granulation tissue should be removed to (0.5 cm) below skin level. Because the epithelium at the periphery of the wound in these chronic cases is usually keratinized and totally quiescent, a 2-mm wide strip should be removed to stimulate resumption of mitotic division. The leading edge of the wound is usually undermined for a distance of 0.5–1.0 cm to encourage epithelial cells while retarding granulation. Pressure bandaging can be used to control hemorrhage. There is no justification for use of caustics, such as copper sulphate, acids, or tissue cauterizants which are non-selective in their action and which will destroy the delicate advancing epithelial margin.

Within 7–10 days fresh granulation tissue will have developed up to skin level and grafting can be considered. Skin grafting is a simple and rewarding procedure (see p. 79). In the event that the granulation tissue returns or is unhealthy either focally or generally, a repeat of this procedure should be contemplated.

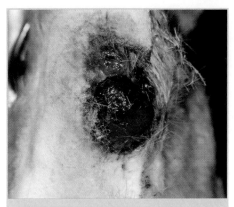

Figure 59 This is an unusual site for excessive granulation tissue, and was due to a bone sequestrum at the site of an old mandibular fracture.

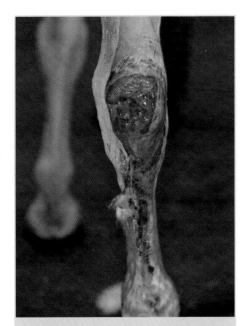

Figure 60 An indolent wound on the plantar hock that shows no significant granulation tissue and yet expanded significantly over a wider area. This is the most common site for this type of response.

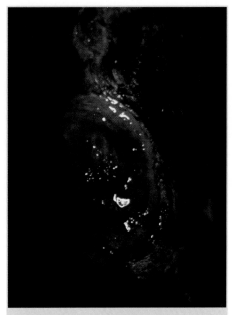

Figure 61 Unhealthy granulation tissue with a spongy edematous nature at the site of a palmar cannon injury. This type of granulation tissue represents an abnormal inflammatory process, and it is important to establish the reasons for this.

Chapter Preview

7 Skin Grafting

Grafting is an effective method for the management of granulation tissue but is not usually suitable for managing cases where there are identifiable reasons for the non-healing of the wound[14].

If the wound is affected by chronic and deep-seated infection or has foreign bodies, sarcoid cells, excessive movement, poor blood supply, an inappropriate pH for healing, or necrotic tissue or impaired blood supply it is unlikely to heal with grafts[15].

Skin grafting should not be attempted until the wound is in a suitably healthy state. It is sometimes possible to divide a wound site into healthy and unhealthy areas. The former can be grafted while the latter is managed to restore a healthy bed of granulation tissue free of infection or clefting.

Free skin grafts should be considered in situations when there is a full thickness skin deficits, epithelialization is not active or is retarded, and when wound contraction is not occurring. Grafting should also be considered when conventional suturing techniques and sliding flaps are not possible; large defects below the carpus and hock frequently fall into this category. Spontaneous healing in these cases will be protracted and often results finally in dense (cheloid or hypertrophic) scar (see p. 89).

Skin grafting can result in a more cosmetic and functional scar than would result from second intention healing. It can also improve wound healing with fewer functional problems, shorten recuperation time, and decrease the chance of long-term medical problems which in turn decreases the need for long-term nursing care. Grafts incur positive cost–benefit, as long-term wound management is one of the most expensive procedures.

Classification of Grafts

Grafts are classified according to the donor–recipient relationship and the thickness/shape of the graft skin. The accepted classification includes:
1. Autograft: tissue is taken from the animal itself.
2. Allograft (homograft): tissue is taken from the same species but a different animal.
3. Xenograft (heterograft): tissue is taken from a different species.

Grafts are also classified according to the thickness of the skin derived from the donor site into pedicle grafts, free skin grafts (full thickness and split skin grafts), and artificial skin replacements.

Pedicle Graft

At least one attachment to the donor site is maintained during healing. Flaps of skin with a broad attachment can sometimes be used to cover difficult wound sites (e.g. eyelid injuries). In some locations it may be possible to use skin stretching (balloon) systems before attempting to perform a pedicle graft. The commonest form of pedicle graft in horses is conjunctival grafting for corneal injuries and ulcerations (Figure 62). There are various forms of flap graft that can be used, including Y- and Z-plasty and tube grafts. These are described in surgical texts.

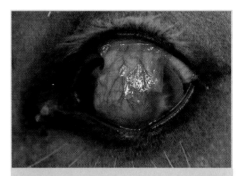

Figure 62 A conjunctival flap (pedicle) graft on an injured cornea 4 weeks postsurgery.

Vascular pedicle grafts are flaps of skin transferred with their intact vascular supply. This is not used significantly in horses yet. Likewise, free vascular pedicle grafts consist of donor skin removed with its major blood vessels, which are anastomosed at the recipient site to convenient local vessels. These are increasingly used in human cosmetic and reconstructive surgery, but not yet in the horse.

Free Grafts

The donor skin is dependent from the outset on the recipient site for its nutrition. There are two main forms that are simply classified in terms of the thickness of the skin graft, and therefore on the extent of adnexal structures. The thinner grafts (split thickness grafts) have no hair follicles, while the thicker ones (full thickness grafts) have intact hair follicles (Figure 63).

Full Thickness Grafts

All elements of epidermis and dermis are retained in full thickness grafts without subcutaneous tissue and fascia. They can only be used to cover a limited area because of the restrictions imposed by the donor site. The major problem with full thickness grafts (of all types) is shearing force between the graft and the recipient bed, and unless the recipient site can be immobilized there is a relatively high failure rate. However, the cosmetic effects are much better because the adnexa are also transferred.

There are several different methods including meshed grafts and 'postage stamp' grafts (modified Meek method). Meshed grafts can be expanded to cover a larger area than the donor area (up to 150% of the original donor site area). Meshing also allows drainage of fluids, an important benefit as accumulation of fluids under grafts is a common cause of failure of non-meshed grafts. The cosmetic effects are better than split skin grafts and pinch grafts because the adnexa survive. Meshed grafts are an all or nothing option: if part of the graft fails then usually it will all fail.

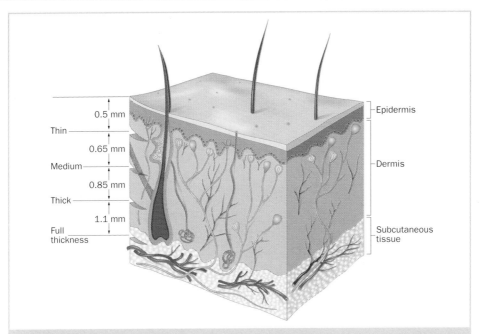

Figure 63 Drawing of skin showing the position of the sectioning of skin for the various skin grafting techniques. (Modified from JA Auer and JA Stick, *Equine Surgery*, 2nd edn, 1999, WB Saunders.)

'Postage stamp' grafts (modified Meek method) uses small squares of skin (usually around 3–5 mm square) attached to an adhesive dressing. A special machine is used for preparation of the squares but simply cutting the skin into small squares could in theory produce suitable donor skin. The method allows the further expansion of the donor area to 1.5–2 times the original. The grafts are not dependent on the survival of all the squares: if a few do not survive they do not affect the others. Cosmetically the results are excellent, but the major disadvantage is the need to ensure the grafts are immobilized. To this end a rigid limb cast is usually applied[16].

Tunnel (Strip) Grafts

Tunnel (strip) grafts can be used when the graft bed is less than ideal. The cosmetic effects are inferior to mesh grafting but the technique is more practical[17]. It requires less time, effort and expertise, and can be performed with minimal equipment in the standing animal. Success is not usually the all or nothing phenomenon associated with mesh grafts.

Narrow strips of donor skin are obtained by parallel incisions 2 mm apart (Figure 64). All subcutaneous tissue is removed with a scalpel. About four or five strips can be obtained from a single site, which is then closed with sutures. The grafts are placed using 8 cm-long alligator forceps with a 2 mm diameter. Starting at the periphery of the wound, the forceps are inserted 5–10 mm deep into the granulation tissue and then passed horizontally through it to emerge on the opposite side. The grafts are drawn through the newly created tunnel. Care is taken not to twist them. The exposed ends are sutured or glued to the skin at the wound margin.

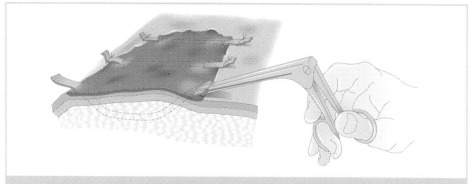

Figure 64 Drawing of the technique for tunnel grafting. In most cases there is no need to bring the grafts to the surface in the middle of the grafted field, but this can help if the granulation tissue is on a curvature.

The site is dressed with a hydrogel and polymeric foam dressing and left for 3–4 days. Dressings are renewed as required. Six to 10 days after surgery the covering granulation tissue can be excised to expose the grafts, but usually some regression of the granulation is obvious by then. The wound is kept covered until epithelialization is complete. Movement is much less significant with this type of graft.

Pinch Grafts

These are the simplest and most practical method and require no special instrumentation. However, the cosmetic effects are sometimes not very acceptable. Split thickness skin in the form of pinch grafts is embedded in the granulation tissue (Figure 65). The procedure can be carried out in the standing horse under sedation using local analgesia at the donor site, or under general anesthesia. The recipient site must be suitable for grafting (see p. 75). The skin is elevated with the tip of a half-curved cutting needle held in needle holders, and a small disc of split thickness skin 3–4 mm in diameter is excised with a No.11 scalpel blade. Twelve to 15 grafts are harvested from a surgically prepared site on the horse's neck or belly at a time and placed into a sterile Petri dish.

The grafts are implanted in the granulation tissue 1 cm apart in a downward direction at an angle of 45° using fine, pointed, plain tissue forceps. *It is wise to start grafting at the most distal part first so that bleeding does not obscure the site for the next row of grafts.* Alternatively, they can be implanted in 'pockets' 1 cm deep created using a No.15 scalpel blade.

The grafts may become dislodged by bleeding in the recipient cup and this may be partially prevented by using a small bleb of tissue adhesive over the entry point or by simply pressing on each site for few seconds.

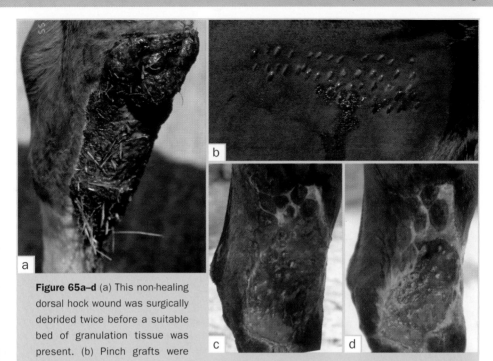

Figure 65a–d (a) This non-healing dorsal hock wound was surgically debrided twice before a suitable bed of granulation tissue was present. (b) Pinch grafts were taken from the neck and buried in the granulation tissue. (c) By 28 days the wound was noticeably smaller and the first grafts were visible as islands of epithelial cells. (d) By 42 days the wound had contracted significantly, and a second grafting was performed. It then went on to heal well. Some hair was present in tufts. (Courtesy of Chris Proudman.)

Note

Punch grafts (Figure 66) are an alternative technique in which full thickness pieces of skin are harvested with a 9 mm skin biopsy punch. The skin punches are then implanted in 6 mm holes created in the granulation tissue with a smaller punch. The recipient holes can be plugged temporarily with cotton swabs until bleeding has reduced. Fibrin 'glue' or cyanomethacrylate tissue adhesive can help to retain the grafts in position.

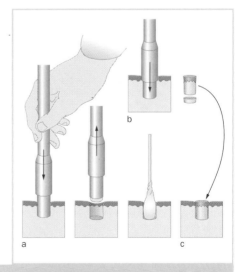

Figure 66a–c (a) Recipient cavities are obtained by using a 6 mm punch biopsy instrument in the granulating bed. The caivities are plugged with a cotton swab. (b) The grafts are obtained using a 9 mm punch from the donor site. (c) The grafts are placed in the wound bed. (Modified from TS Stashak, *Equine Wound Management* 1991, Lea and Febiger.)

The wound is covered with a hydrogel or a paraffin gauze dressing (e.g. Jelonet; Smith and Nephew) and a firm Robert Jones' dressing. Movement will cause some of the grafts to be dislodged, which will be evident when the dressing is changed 3–4 days after grafting. Loss of more than 10% of the grafts is usually associated with poor technique/condition in one or more of: implantation, postoperative management, granulation tissue bed, vascularization, or sarcoid transformation of the wound site.

Usually however, a significant proportion will 'take' and these will be evident as epithelial 'islands' after 3–4 weeks. Successful (viable) grafts have a noticeable effect in controlling granulation tissue and can be recognized by blanching of the granulation tissue bed (usually seen between 7–21 days) as neovascularization is inhibited. More active epithelialization is also seen at the periphery of the wound, and obvious wound contraction is evident around 21–27 days postgrafting. Islands of graft-derived epithelium are visible around 21–35 days, and hair tufts may be visible at around 42–56 days.

Split Thickness Grafts

These can be taken at various cleavage planes so that the graft comprises epidermis and various thicknesses of dermal tissue. The options are thin, intermediate, or thick. Sheets of split thickness skin can be harvested with a dermatome, usually 0.7 mm thick is most appropriate in horses. Split thickness grafts may be taken from the ventral abdomen, brisket/chest, ischial region, or side of the neck. It may be used as a sheet over the whole wound or as a mesh graft produced by running it through a mesh dermatome, which produces multiple small parallel staggered cuts to allow expansion of the graft . This will usually allow an expansion to a maximum of 150%.

The graft is cut to overlap the edges of the recipient site by 1.5 cm, and is sutured to the skin with 3/0 monofilament nylon, or alternatively fixed to the *skin* with n-butyl methacrylate tissue adhesives ('Superglue'). A tie-over pack is used to maintain contact of the graft with the granulation tissue bed. Any tendency for exudate to accumulate under the graft can be minimized by making a number of small incisions in the graft, and ensuring even pressure by the tie-over pack dressing.

The Meek technique permits greater expansion of the donor site (up to 400%) and is a useful if cumbersome method that can also be used with split skin (see p. 80).

Mesh Split Skin Grafts (Figures 67, 68)

Mesh grafts are said to provide the best functional and cosmetic outcomes but have several disadvantages[18]. They are best harvested with a dermatome and meshed with a mesh expander; both are expensive pieces of equipment. As for the full thickness skin mesh grafts, failure is common when split skin mesh grafts are used in less than ideal locations, e.g. over the dorsal aspect of the hock.

If part of the mesh starts to fail, failure of the entire graft usually follows. The patient must be anesthetized for the graft to be harvested and applied. Cosmetically the results are less satisfactory because the hair follicles are not usually included, but the thinner graft and exposure of more of the stratum germanitivum means that the 'take' may be better than with full thickness grafts.

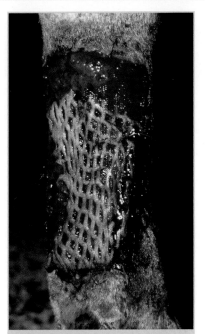

Figure 67 A meshed split skin graft being applied to a wound with healthy granulation tissue. (Courtesy of J Schumacher.)

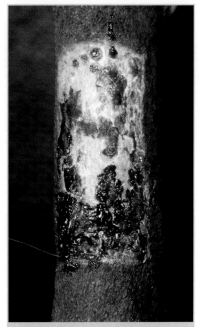

Figure 68 The appearance of the graft site in Figure 67 49 days postsurgery. (Courtesy of J Schumacher.)

Artificial Skin Substitutes/Replacements

A number of new approaches have developed out of the need to obtain an artificial source of a skin substitute for patients with extensive skin loss and few useful donor skin sites. The possibilities include autogenous cultured keratinocytes laid on the wound surface, and a sterile dressing comprising dermal cells in a collagen-based matrix. These are not available for horses at present, but it is likely that in the future the technology will be applicable.

Clinico-pathological Consequences of Grafting

Grafts encourage contraction; the location of the donor site appears to be a significant factor in the contraction at the recipient site. They also stimulate local epithelialization in addition to producing their own epithelium.

Grafts also inhibit formation of excess granulation tissue (see p. 75); the effect will be noticeable in grafted wounds within days of surgery. A wound that has been grafted will be seen to 'blanch' after about 7–21 days as the blood supply is reduced. An additional benefit in using grafting is in the control of wound infection and inflammation; a decline in the number of bacteria in the graft–bed interface and in granulation tissue has been demonstrated shortly after grafting[19].

Graft Take and Causes of Failure

Graft 'take' or survival depends on the establishment of adequate vascular connections between the graft and the recipient bed acceptance, and takes place in several defined phases: adherence, plasmatic imbibition, and revascularization, shown in Figure 69.

In the adherence phase, initially the graft is held in place by fibrin exuded from the wound, and receives temporary nutrition through plasmatic imbibition; the contracted, empty vessels dilate and passively absorb serum, which percolates through the fibrin meshwork. This fluid does not circulate and the graft consequently appears cyanotic until revascularization takes place. Revascularization only occurs when there is close and stable graft–bed contact.

There are three mechanisms of revascularization, which begin 24–28 hours after grafting: host vessels anastomose with graft vessels (inosculation); capillary buds from the host penetrate into the existing vascular system of the graft using the old vessels as conduits; and capillary buds construct a completely new vascular system in the graft.

Organization

Fibroblasts infiltrate the fibrin around the graft site within 72 hours after transplantation, and slowly produce fibrous adhesions. These fibrous adhesions and functional vessels traversing the graft–bed interface result in a firm attachment of the graft within 9–10 days of grafting. Wound contraction, pigmentation and reinnervation may take up to 18 months to complete.

A successful outcome is most likely when the graft is placed on healthy, non-infected, convex shaped, immobile granulation tissue, or on a fresh wound surface.

Note

Grafts will not take on avascular sites, e.g. denuded bones without periosteum, bared tendon without paratenon, or cartilage surfaces without perichondrium. In addition, grafts will not take on infected tissue, sarcoid tissue, or on other poor recipient beds including fat, heavily irradiated tissue, old granulation tissue, irregular granulation tissue, and surfaces with chronic ulceration.

Causes of Graft Failure

The most common reasons for graft failure are:
1. Poor graft harvesting technique.
2. Poor recipient bed.
3. Infection.
4. Hematoma and seroma under the graft.
5. Movement of the graft relative to the recipient site (shear forces).
6. Poor blood supply to the graft bed.
7. Tumor transformation (sarcoid).

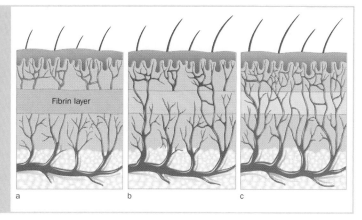

Figure 69 Representation of the mechanism of graft take. (a) Adherence, plasmatic imbibition, (b) inosculation, (c) revascularization. (Modified from JA Auer and JA Stick, *Equine Surgery*, 2nd edn, 1999, WB Saunders.)

Fibrin layer

a   b   c

Wound Preparation and Timing of Grafting

Grafting requires preparation and after care. Fresh traumatic wounds can rarely be grafted and the wound is only ready for grafting when there is a healthy bed of young red granulation tissue, which bleeds readily when wiped with a dry swab, has minimal discharge, and has a smooth contour appropriate to the surrounding skin. A healthy bed of granulation devoid of infection is absolutely essential for full thickness or split thickness sheet grafts, but is slightly less important if pinch, punch, or tunnel grafts are used.

Preparation of the Recipient Site

If granulation tissue is excessive (see p. 75), it should be excised to 0.5 cm below skin level, and a sterile non-adhesive dressing and pressure bandage applied (see p. 61). The dressing should be replaced at 48 hour intervals until smooth pink granulation tissue is present which is slightly 'proud'; it may take up to 7–10 days.

During the 24 hours prior to grafting, covering the wound with gauze which is then repeatedly soaked in saline and allowed to dry prior to removal, is an effective method of ensuring a clean surface to the granulation tissue. Application of a steroid-based water soluble cream over the last 24–48 hours may help considerably. The hair should be clipped for some distance from the wound edges, and the area washed thoroughly and rinsed with saline (spirit washes are not advised).

Summary

The successful use of skin grafts requires some experience and depends on the appropriate choice of graft type, meticulous wound and graft preparation, and careful application and postoperative care. Although movement can be a major disrupting factor in all types of graft, the use of casts can present problems, which may exceed the benefits achieved by rigid immobilization. Grafting can be a very rewarding procedure with a rapid return to health, and should be considered early in the management of wounds likely to be complicated by prolonged healing or where there is a significant skin deficit.

Chapter Preview

8 Dealing with Scar Tissue

Scarring is an inevitable consequence of injury. Not every horse will heal with fine or insignificant scars. The extent and type of scarring is dependent on the extent of the wound, the anatomical location of the wound, and the presence or absence of complicating factors (with the wound itself or surrounding structures). In addition, the duration of the inflammatory response (including the time between injury and the first proper examination) and the individual characteristics of healing of the horse (size, breed, and health status) will affect scarring.

Because reduction of a scar is extremely difficult it is important to minimize the extent of scarring by good wound management in the first instance. Normal scarring restores up to 80% of the original tensile strength and is always recognizable histologically. Scars usually contract with time. Inappropriate or extensive scarring is more common when second intention healing takes place and on limb wounds of larger horses.

Consequences of Scarring

Scarring resulting from tissue loss can result in functional deficits. For instance, damage to vital structures, such as the cornea, brain, or major motor nerves can significantly impair normal function. Functional loss can also occur from involvement of vital structures in the scar; fortunately equine scarring is not accompanied by serious contraction and so presents fewer functional problems than in some other species such as the human. However, scar contraction/cicatrization in delicate skin structures such as the eyelids can be functionally catastrophic or functionally limiting (such as in the mouth or nostril).

Deformity or hair loss and (often) changes in color of the skin and hair are sometimes unacceptable to the owner, e.g. in a show horse, but are unavoidable. Careful attention to detail during healing may limit the cosmetic effects.

Types of Scar

The type and extent of scarring is unpredictable in horses; some wounds heal remarkably well (see p. 17) while others heal inappropriately with abnormal scar formation.

Normal Scar

In a normal scar functional deficits are minimal with close restoration of normal tissue anatomy and minimal cosmetic effects. The scar is smaller than the original wound and scar contraction continues after healing has been completed.

Abnormal Scar

Hypertrophic scarring

In hypertrophic scarring the scar is larger than the original wound (Figure 70) as the scar continues to expand. There is dense fibrosis and high blood supply, and the scar is not usually fragile nor easily traumatized.

Cheloid Scarring

A cheloid scar is larger than the original wound and usually static in size (Figure 71), and is thickened, rough, and has a hyperkeratotic 'reptilian' appearance. There is increased blood supply, and the scar is fragile and easily traumatized.

Weak/Fragile Scarring

The scar is thin and vascular with poor epithelial cover and is easily traumatized. It lacks tensile strength and the wound site can easily be distracted.

Limiting the Severity of Scarring

The best policy for scar management has to be the limitation of the extent of the scar in the first place. Wounds that heal slowly produce more scar tissue and this is less controllable. Best practice wound management and limiting the chronic inflammatory process are the main factors required. Corticosteroid ointments applied topically may help at some sites, e.g. the cornea. Scarring can, in theory, be reduced by direct application or injection of neutralizing antibody to transforming growth factor-beta (TGF-β)[20].

Cheloid and hypertrophic scarring may relate to specific events in the chronic inflammatory process but may be genetically programmed (i.e. certain families of horse are more prone to poor or inappropriate scar formation). The health and nutritional status of the patient is important: healthy animals heal faster and better than unhealthy ones and with less scar. Deficiencies in specific nutritional factors, e.g. zinc and vitamins A and C may lead to abnormal scarring.

Management of Scar Tissue

Surgical excision is the only way to eliminate existent densely fibrotic scar tissue, but the consequences may be even worse than the original scar. There is always the danger that the surgical wound will in fact heal poorly so that the scar is as bad or even worse than the original. Surgery can, however, be useful in severely compromising scarring, such as in intestinal and esophageal circumferential scarring. Surgery is performed under ideal elective conditions with healthy tissues and so postoperative scarring can be less prominent.

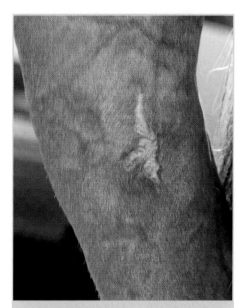

Figure 70 A hypertrophic scar. This scar developed at the site of a very small wound. The horse suffered from similar problems at all sites of wounding.

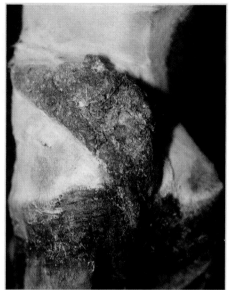

Figure 71 This cheloid scar was fragile and easily damaged. The healing tissue has a distinctly reptilian appearance. Healing followed surgical removal of all the abnormal tissue and the application of moist wound management methods. Grafting was not necessary.

Removal of a scarred area of skin followed by grafting (flap or pedicle graft or free skin grafts, see p. 79) is possibly the best surgical method of scar treatment. The rate of failure is high and the procedure is difficult and expensive.

Keratolytic preparations, e.g. coal tar ointments, reduce the thickness of the epithelial cells over the scar and so it might appear to be a softer and suppler tissue.

Scar management with hydrating silicone dressings (CicaCare; Smith and Nephew) is a new method of managing skin scars but has limitations. The silicone sheet has to be retained in contact with the scar for as long as possible (weeks or months). Retaining the sheet in position may cause skin injury that may be worse than the original problem! It is not appropriate for fresh wounds or fresh scars, and is most useful for mature scars. The dressing is applied to the scarred area and maintained in contact for as many hours per day as possible. A (Pressage) elasticized bandage may be useful for this if the scar is on the tarsus or carpus.

Natural substances such as alovera and arnica have been used topically and by mouth but there is no proof of efficacy. Homeopathic remedies are totally unproven. Those who sell them view them as a positive aid.

Section 4
Management of Complicated Wounds

Chapter Preview

▶ Skin Lacerations with Skin Deficits or Degloving

▶ Wounds Involving Muscle Damage

▶ Wounds Involving Synovial Structures

▶ Wounds with Exposed bone

▶ Eyelid Injuries

▶ Eye Injuries

▶ Wounds Involving the Mouth, Tongue and Jaws

▶ Wounds Involving Nerve Damage

▶ Wounds Involving Cranial Damage

▶ Wounds Involving Hoof Capsule and Coronary Band

▶ Wounds Involving Open Body Cavities

▶ Wounds Involving Major Blood Vessels

9 Complicated Wounds

Wounds that are correctly examined and treated at an early stage have a much higher chance of healing quickly and with minimal complications. Wounds that are neglected or managed badly, regardless of their severity or otherwise, will inevitably heal poorly, slowly, and with more extensive scarring. The rate and efficiency of wound healing largely depends upon factors such as site, complications, inhibitors of healing, time between wounding and treatment, and the type of treatment applied.

Recent research has confirmed that certain areas on the horse heal better than others, and that ponies tend to heal better than horses[1]. Body wounds on horses and ponies usually heal remarkably well with a high element of contraction, and leave scars that are much smaller than the original wound. Limb wounds on large horses heal notoriously badly and tend to heal by epithelialization and scars may be larger than the original wound. The worst region for healing is the distal limb region (both fore and hind) of horses over 145 cm. Limb wounds of ponies (<145 cm) heal as well as wounds on the trunk of larger horses and healing is particularly impressive on the trunk of ponies[12].

Most complicated wounds involve several tissue types; where this is so, the wound must be assessed carefully so that measures are taken to deal with the most urgent problems first. There is no point in closing a skin wound while the deeper tissues remain seriously injured and unlikely to heal.

The presence or absence of factors that inhibit or retard healing will affect scarring (see p. 25). Early physiologically sound treatment provides the best chance of healing (even for difficult or complicated wounds). Neglected/long-standing (chronic) wounds become progressively less likely to heal with passing time.

Poor wound management hinders healing, while a 'gold standard' approach provides the best chances for rapid healing with minimal scarring and functional deficits. Every effort should be made to use only physiologically sound procedures and meticulous surgical management. Modern wound dressings play an active role in wound healing, and should be selected specifically for each stage of the healing process of every individual wound.

Skin Lacerations with Deficits of Degloving

Introduction

Skin injuries with skin deficits and/or 'degloving' are relatively common (Figures 72, 73), and management of these injuries can be very difficult. The absence of 'spare' (loose) skin on limbs means that large deficits in these sites require particular care. Notwithstanding the best possible care, healing is likely to be prolonged.

Degloving injuries are commonest on the upper limb regions; the skin on the lower limb is probably more firmly attached and seldom 'degloves' in the same way as the upper limb and body trunk. These injuries should be treated promptly to restore as much of the skin as possible to its original position (even if it is probably non-viable). Degloving of limbs usually involves at least some horizontal skin laceration and is usually in a downward direction so that the skin hangs around the limb.

The exposed subcutaneous tissues rapidly become dry and infected but remarkably little bleeding occurs in most such cases. The blood supply to the upper margin of the wound is usually intact and so this is less of a problem than the distal wound margin, which is invariably compromised – especially at the most central part of the wound margin. Sloughing of the skin along this margin is common.

Preliminary Approach

The wound should be irrigated with copious warm sterile saline and protected from further contamination by application of a hydrogel to the exposed tissues. This will minimize dehydration and infection. The flap should be restored to its natural position as far as possible, and bandaged onto the site if practicable until a more detailed examination can be performed. This maintains warmth, prevents further contamination and devitalization, and covers the exposed tissues with a biological dressing.

Movement of the limb should be minimized so that tension on the wound is reduced as far as possible. Shear forces will be maximal during movement of the underlying muscles relative to the skin. Large skin deficits should initially be dressed with a hydrogel after warm saline irrigation. There is seldom any spare skin that can be mobilized, and so a prolonged recovery and/or extensive surgical procedures may be expected.

Surgical Procedure

The wound should be carefully examined (possibly even under general anesthesia) and, after superficial irrigation, all obvious foreign matter and devitalized subcutaneous tissues scrupulously removed. Deeper injuries are treated accordingly by lavage, and if indicated by suturing the defects with an absorbable suture material of suitable diameter and pattern. Skin should not be removed unless it is totally devitalized and shredded.

Carefully placed subcutaneous 'walking sutures' limit dead space by firmly fixing the skin to the deeper structures, but this may not always be possible. This minimizes tension on any single part

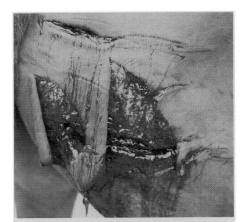

Figure 72 Extensive skin lacerations with skin deficits from a road traffic accident. The injury healed well by second intention, although initially the skin was sutured where possible to reduce the healing time.

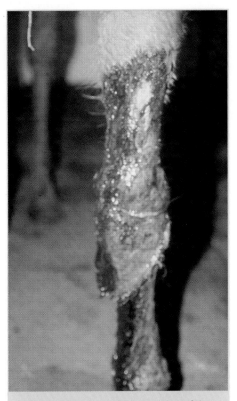

Figure 73 A severe degloving injury of the forearm. Walking sutures and drains were used to restore the skin approximately to normal position, but the wound broke down extensively and took some months to heal by second intention. (Courtesy of RR Pascoe.)

of the incision; with careful extension of the skin it may be possible to eliminate tension on the wound line. If the injury is more than 1–2 hours old, the skin will have shrunk significantly, and it may be difficult to restore it to its natural position. The skin wound is closed using interrupted horizontal or vertical mattress sutures with monofilament nylon (4 or 5 metric/1 or 2 USP). Tension across the wound site can be relieved by supported quill sutures.

If there is deep tissue disruption, fluid accumulation must be prevented. A surgical drain exiting the wound below its most dependent aspect is helpful (this may involve a separate skin incision). Firm dressings can be used to apply direct pressure but this must be controlled carefully to prevent further compromise of the cutaneous vasculature. Alternatively the wound can be left partially closed so that fluid can drain freely.

Follow-up Measures

Movement should be restricted depending on the extent and type of wound.

Dressings should be changed as and when indicated. Variable necrosis of at least part of the skin margin is commonly present. In any case, the necrotic tissue will eventually need to be removed and the wound allowed to heal by second intention or by some form of grafting.

Wounds Involving Muscle Damage

Introduction

These wounds involve the upper limb or body trunk regions (Figure 74). Wounds involving muscle damage sometimes bleed quite heavily – this is particularly so if the muscle is lacerated (as opposed to bruised or crushed).

Large flap wounds involving extensive skin and muscle damage are common in horses, particularly when the injury occurs at speed.

Wounds caused by sharp objects (e.g. glass, metal, or sharp plastic) tend to be almost surgical with little maceration but may have multiple lacerations. Those involving kicks or

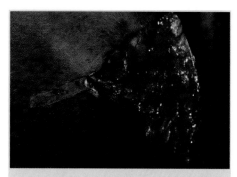

Figure 74 A deep laceration with muscle involvement. The wound was repaired in three layers and healed by primary union.

falls at speed are complicated by extensive skin avulsion and deep muscular bruising with laceration and damage. In the case of barbed wire wounds, the edges are often ragged and there may be several cuts in close proximity to one another.

At this stage it may not be possible to decide which tissue is viable. Many extensive wounds that are left to heal by second intention heal largely by contraction. Cosmetic results tend to be good with a significantly smaller scar than the wound (see p. 17). Primary closure of the muscle deficits may shorten the recovery period and improve functional restoration. Fresh injuries are far more amenable to primary closure. The location of the wound is important because muscle damage may be more important over the eyes or on the face than on major muscle masses.

There may be moderate or severe skin deficits that will need to be considered at an early stage. Discoloration of the underlying muscle may be indicative of serious compromise: dark or black muscle may be non-viable or severely desiccated, whereas bright red active muscle is likely to have a good blood supply (there may be more bleeding in this case). Any delays in restoration of the skin to its normal position will result in shrinkage and reduced viability of the flap.

Preliminary Approach

Adequate restraint should be used to permit close examination, which may require sedation with an α-2-agonist (e.g. romifidine, detomidine, xylazine) (see p. 39). Hemorrhage should be controlled (see p. 39), and appropriate anesthesia (regional blocks or local inverted L block) is required for exploration, cleaning, and possible suturing. Local anesthetic infiltration into the wound itself is not conducive to healing, and should be avoided if possible by using regional blocks. In particular, anesthetic with adrenaline should not be used.

The wound should immediately be covered with a hydrogel and the margins of the wound carefully clipped or shaven to establish the full extent of the injury, and in particular the full extent of the underlying muscle damage. The skin flap and the underlying muscles should be handled gently and washed carefully with warm saline. Chemical antiseptics should be avoided as far as possible unless there is gross contamination. Antibiotic powders (such as crystalline penicillin and aureomycin powder) may be cytotoxic and therefore retard healing. If the wound is infected or is likely to be infected then such an approach may be helpful, i.e. the benefit outweighs the disadvantages. The wound should be irrigated with copious warm (body temperature) sterile saline (as much as the horse will allow) to remove superficial contamination and the residues of the hydrogel. Further applications of hydrogel to the wound site will keep the surface moist and protected against further bacterial contamination.

No skin should be removed if at all possible. Replacing the skin into its natural position temporarily will keep it warm, and will provide a biological cover for the underlying muscles so that they will not dry out or become injured further.

Surgical Procedure

All foreign matter and necrotic/nonviable/compromised tissue should be removed from the wound bed by sharp excision (using a scalpel rather than scissors). Assuming that the wound is surgically clean, the deeper layers of muscle are closed carefully with 1 or 2 metric polyglactin (e.g. Vicryl), using a mattress or simple continuous suture pattern.

The skin should be restored to its natural position, although this may be difficult due to shrinkage if there have been any delays. Walking sutures placed subcutaneously between the skin and the underlying muscles are useful in reducing the dead space, ensuring that the skin is firmly placed up against the underlying muscle, reducing the tension on the suture line, and reducing the extent of skin shrinkage/contraction.

If there is extensive muscle bruising and possible necrosis a surgical drain should be inserted. A latex Penrose capillary drain can be used with its exit at a specially made exit portal at or below the most dependent part of the wound.

Vacuum drains can also be useful provided that they can be maintained. Fenestrated tube drains are useful in allowing the wound to be flushed but rapidly block-up and become useless.

The skin wound is closed using either horizontal mattress sutures (if the tension is mild), vertical mattress sutures (where cosmesis is important and tension is mild), simple interrupted sutures (where tension is not significant), or supported quill tension sutures (where tension is high).

A stent made from gauze swabs covered in hydrogel can be used to cover the wound, and serves both as a protection and a means of reducing the tension on the suture line. Dressings are applied over the wound if convenient. Non-steroidal anti-inflammatory drug (e.g. telzenac, phenylbutazone, or ketoprofen) are useful to reduce inflammatory responses and provide analgesia. Pain can be controlled by opioid analgesics such as butorphanol. Antibiotics are advisable and penicillin is probably the antibiotic of choice. It is unlikely that areas with large blocks of underlying muscle will be amenable to bandaging.

> **Note**
>
> If there is extensive muscle loss and destruction the wound can safely be left to heal by second intention, but must be managed carefully to maintain a sustained contraction and healing. It is remarkable how even extensive body wounds involving major muscle damage will heal without apparent problems and minimal cosmetic effects and functional difficulties.

Follow-up Measures

Dressings should be changed at appropriate intervals. If there is significant exudate consider more frequent changes and/or the use of a high volume absorbent dressing (e.g. a disposable nappy). If the wound is clean and non-exudative there is usually no extra value in repeated dressings. Intervals of up to 3–5 days are possible if modern wound dressings and hydrogels are used. The tetanus status of the horse should be checked, and toxoid given if there is unknown vaccination history but the horse is known to have been vaccinated, or tetanus antiserum when there is unknown, uncertain, or no previous vaccination.

Wounds Involving Synovial Structures

Introduction

Wounds resulting in penetration of any synovial structure can lead to life threatening infection and extreme lameness and should be treated as an emergency. All joint injuries are serious, and must be recognized at the outset as delay in treatment is potentially catastrophic. Injuries over 12 hours old usually carry a poor prognosis, while those over 24 hours have an almost hopeless prognosis.

Not all wounds extend perpendicularly into the deeper structures and so the skin wound may not directly overlie a joint (Figure 75). Deficits of the joint capsule are a serious complication (Figure 76). Some injuries involving joints or tendons are complicated by fractures. Injuries involving the flexor tendons during full limb extension (i.e. the tendon is at full tension) cause severe damage (or even total disruption). The skin injury may appear to be relatively trivial (Figure 77). Furthermore, the tendon injury may be at a site that is quite a distance from the skin injury. The exact location and extent of the wound should be established.

Careful radiographic and ultrasonographic examinations are essential. Synovial fluid leakage may be obvious or may be difficult to identify; clear yellow, somewhat oily fluid exuding from the depth of the wound could be joint fluid, but the difference between serum exudate and synovial fluid is not always clear, especially when there is some inflammation of the joint that results in a cloudy synovial fluid that lacks normal viscosity. No wound that has synovial fluid drainage should be trivialized or left untreated.

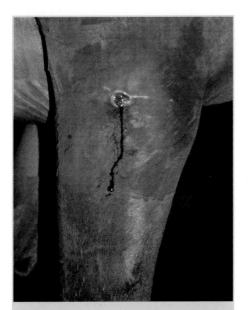

Figure 75 The lateral pouch of the elbow joint is frequently well away from the apparent site of the elbow itself. This small wound gave no real indication of the severity of the problem.

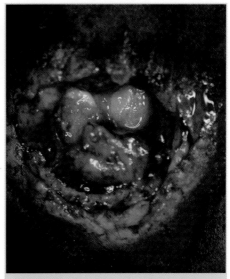

Figure 76 Severe abrasion of the fetlock joint from a trailer injury. Although the injury is particularly severe with extensive tissue loss, immediate treatment resulted in a surprisingly satisfactory repair after some months.

Close observation of the posture of the foot and fetlock when the horse is made to take weight on the leg will help to identify tendon disruption.

Severance of the superficial digital flexor tendon produces only slight dropping of the fetlock, whereas deep digital flexor severance results in toe lifting from the ground and is extremely serious; this is unlikely in a wound without superficial flexor tendon damage. Complete disruption of the suspensory apparatus results in a dropped fetlock and lifted toe. Although disruption of the extensor tendon initially results in knuckling over at the fetlock, the horse quickly adapts. Normal function may be restored as the tendon ends become incorporated in the granulation tissue.

The cause of the wound is a useful factor in deciding on the likely treatment.

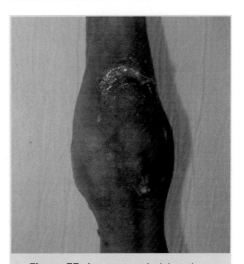

Figure 77 An over-reach injury in a racehorse. The location of the injury suggests that the digital sheath was involved. With emergency treatment the wound healed without complication.

Sharp lacerations are usually easier to repair than those complicated by extensive tissue bruising and widespread damage to adjacent structures. If the patient cannot move or is unwilling to move there may be concurrent damage to other structures (joints/bones). The horse should not be moved (an ambulance or trailer may be helpful) as movement can exacerbate a tendon or joint injury and may also cause displacement of fractures. It can also result in dissemination of infection. Significant bleeding is unusual.

Preliminary Approach

The wound site should be packed with hydrogel to prevent ingress of further foreign matter, followed by digital exploration of the wound to assess the full range of injuries. Local anesthesia may be required (regional blocks are far better than local infiltration).

Antibiotics and non-steroidal anti-inflammatory drugs (e.g. phenylbutazone) should be administered parenterally at an early stage. *Infection is one of the most dangerous complications of synovial injuries*, and intravenous penicillin and gentamicin is probably the best initial combination. If the joint or tendon sheath is open it may be possible to flush the wound using large volumes of saline. The sterile end of a giving set may be introduced directly into the wound as a first aid measure to flush away gross debris and infective organisms.

A hydrogel is then applied to the wound site and a polymeric foam dressing applied. A full Robert Jones' bandage can be used to limit movement at the wound site. If there is much synovial exudate an absorptive dressing can be used (e.g. a disposable nappy). The horse is then admitted to hospital or referral center for joint/sheath flushing and repair. (*This is a specialist procedure.*)

Surgical Procedure

Most tendon and joint injuries require general anesthesia for full investigation and repair. The wound may have to be enlarged to allow proper assessment and removal of all foreign matter, damaged and non-viable tissue. Copious flushing (usually from a remote site in the synovial structure, via high pressure systems delivering warm saline) helps to remove foreign matter and bacteria. The final flush should be with a suitable antibiotic solution such as gentamicin solution.

Antibiotic impregnated beads may be used within the structure.

The tissues are reconstructed appropriately; flexor tendons may require prosthetic reconstruction. Drains with continuous flushing mechanism to allow continuous flush after recovery are helpful. The decision to close the wound (primary union) or partially close it or leave it open is a matter for the surgeon.

In many cases a delayed primary union is a useful technique provided that further contamination can be prevented. A rigid limb cast may be required once all infection has been controlled.

Follow-up Measures

Suitable supportive shoes should be applied to assist recovery and avoid excessive forces on the healing site. This may be far more difficult than it seems. For example, simply raising the heel transfers forces away from the deep to the superficial flexor tendon. Axial loading has become common practice but this may be problematical in the long-term, and subsequent wound contraction may result in an intractable tendon contracture.

Sustained broad spectrum combination antibiotics are obligatory. Courses of gentamicin or amikacin and crystalline benzylpenicillin are used, but others may be used according to the suspected or proven infective organisms. Repeated synoviocentesis may be indicated, but this should be performed with care and only when useful information can be gained; there is no merit in sampling when the horse shows no pain and is apparently improving clinically.

Drains should be removed as soon as possible. Supportive bandaging and frog supports should be applied to the contralateral limb. The horses should be strictly confined and then given limited exercise in the later stages of healing. Even with the best treatment there is a high rate of complication, and delays of even 4–8 hours may be catastrophic. Owners may not readily appreciate the severity of the injury (particularly of the flexor tendons).

Wounds with Exposed Bone

Introduction

Exposure of bone occurs most often on the distal limb and the face/head (Figure 78). Sequestrum formation occurs when there are fragments of non-viable bone, the periosteum is stripped from the bone, or the periosteum is dried/ desiccated. The blood supply to the bone is disrupted, and the outer one-third of the cortex becomes necrotic because it derives its blood supply from the periosteum. Sequestrum formation also occurs when the exposed surface of the bone is infected.

Sequestrum formation often takes several weeks; the necrotic bone is often obscured by unhealthy granulation tissue.

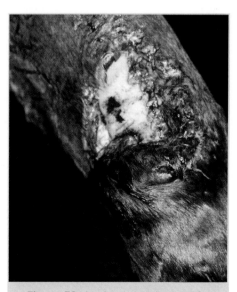

Figure 78 A wire laceration on the forearm in which periosteum was exposed and damaged. The areas of denuded bone formed a sequestrum over the following 12 weeks. Healing was delayed until the necrotic bone had been removed.

Sequestrum can usually be identified radiographically provided the beam is angled appropriately. Sequestration is not an inevitable consequence of periosteal injury, but is a common feature of those wounds that involve periosteal damage that fail to heal. Grafts will not take on denuded bone.

Preliminary Approach

Wounds with exposed bone may be complicated by open joints (see above). Injuries to the lower limb tend to be more dangerous with respect to bone/periosteal damage. Injuries that occur from sharp lacerations tend to induce minimal periosteal damage, whereas injuries that are severely torn or macerated (e.g. barbed wire wounds) tend to produce extensive periosteal damage. Bleeding is usually minimal. Obvious distortion of the bone suggests that there is a concurrent fracture, and open fractures carry a poor or hopeless prognosis. The horse should not be moved without veterinary advice. A firm hydrogel dressing should be applied before transport.

The extent of concurrent soft tissue damage is then assessed, and the area of bone involved determined, including the possibility of fractures (either partial or non-displaced). Immediate radiography may be necessary to eliminate fracture.

If there is no fracture a moist wound dressing (hydrogel and a conformable absorptive dressing) should be applied and a firm bandage used to provide warmth and support. If there is a possibility of a fracture or tendon or joint involvement, a suitable splint can be placed.

Surgical Procedure

Further damage and drying of the periosteum is prevented by application of a hydrogel. The surrounding skin should be clipped and cleaned carefully to expose the full extent of the wound. The wound is flushed with warm sterile normal saline (possibly with 0.5% chlorhexidine solution), and any obvious debris or foreign matter removed. The wound is explored digitally with sterile gloves to establish the extent of the injury and the extent of periosteal damage. Attention should be paid to adjacent synovial structures, tendons, and ligaments. Examination of the wound should also determine the presence of any bony fragments or palpable foreign bodies. The wound is left to granulate while the sequestrum separates.

Follow-up Measures

Healing will be delayed until the sequestrum has formed and been removed (either naturally or surgically) from the wound bed. Radiographs will only show the presence of the developing sequestrum (often as an attached involucrum at first) after 2–4 weeks. Regular follow-up radiographs should be taken at 2–3 week intervals. Dressings should be changed at regular intervals, but there is little to be gained by over-frequent dressings. The degree and the character of any exudate will dictate the interval.

Infection must be controlled. An initial course of 5 days of penicillin can be followed by a prolonged course of trimethoprim sulphur oral powders (or paste). Alternatively, 5-day courses of antibiotics can be given at intervals through the recovery stages. Once confirmed, the sequestrum is located and removed by excising the overlying granulation tissue, and the area is curetted to eliminate any residual infected material. It is extremely unwise to try to dislodge a developing sequestrum by chiseling the bone surface. There is a serious risk of fracture either during surgery or during recovery. Most specialists recover the horse in a rigid limb splint to avoid possible complications.

Eyelid Injuries

Introduction

Eyelid injuries are relatively common in horses. Upper lid injuries have a more profound prognostic implication than injuries to the lower lid because the upper lid performs 76% of the blink function (Figures 79–81). Scarring and deformity can have long-term harmful effects on eye function. Anatomical knowledge is essential if lid function is to be restored. Injury to the nasal quarter of the upper and lower lids can involve the palpebral lacrimal punctae and/or the lacrimal duct. Damage can result in secondary problems of epiphora and facial excoriation.

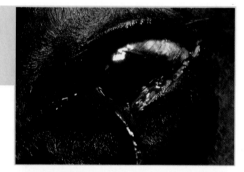

Figure 79 Lower lid laceration that healed well after meticulous reconstruction. This has fewer implications for function than injuries to the upper lid.

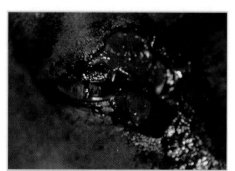

Figure 80 Severe damage to the upper eyelid that involved fractures of the orbital rim. All damaged subcutaneous tissue was removed, and the muscles restored to their natural positions.

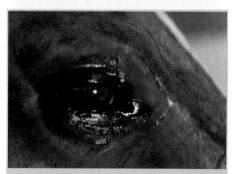

Figure 81 The repair in Figure 80 healed well with an excellent outcome.

Examination of a painful eye can be facilitated by an auriculopalpebral (motor) nerve block inducing upper lid paralysis, or a frontal (sensory) nerve block to anesthetize the upper lid. Local analgesia of the lower lid is much more problematical and involves multiple injections along the eyelid margins where the lacrimal and palpebral nerves are located.

Preliminary Approach

If the eye is involved (or is possibly involved) extra precautions must be taken immediately. There is no point treating the skin wound when this might involve further damaging a dangerously injured eye. Under no circumstances should the eye be pressed during examination – this can result in catastrophic exacerbation of eye injury (see p. 110).

Treatment of upper lid injuries (or more particularly those that are complicated by involvement of the lateral or medial canthus) is more difficult than lower lid injuries.

The extent and depth of skin injury and any skin deficits should be assessed. *Skin flaps must not be cut off under any circumstances*. Early recognition of skin deficits allows rapid reconstructive measures to be performed, thus minimizing the secondary effects on the eye itself.

Parenteral antibiotics can be given: penicillin is probably the most useful, or topical antibiotic drops or ointment (gentamicin or choramphenicol is probably best). Non-steroidal anti-inflammatory drugs (e.g. telzenac, phenylbutazone, or ketoprofen) are useful to reduce the inflammatory process. Reflex or traumatic uveitis is common and can be very painful; this will be relieved by NSAIDs and topical 2% atropine as a mydriatic. Opioid analgesics such as butorphanol may be helpful. If the horse is inclined to self-trauma, sedation with an α-2 agonist (e.g. romifidine, detomidine, xylazine) is indicated.

The skin flap is protected with hydrogel, and the face dressed with a dressing and a protective bandage. The flap should be kept warm by restoring its approximate position, and the cornea protected from injury or drying by the application of artificial tears (e.g. Viscotears). If there is extensive bruising *but no eye damage* consider ice packs (protected by a saline-soaked, soft cotton sheet or flannel).

Note

Proprietary ice packs frozen at −25° to −30°C are probably too cold and should be avoided at this site at this stage. The blood supply to the flap must be preserved and supported.

If the injury causes continued tear leakage, a bandage contact lens can be applied to protect the cornea from rapid drying and damage from inadequate blink responses. The horse should then be moved to a hospital or referral center.

> **Note**
>
> **It is very unwise to attempt repair of the eyelid under sedation and local anesthesia. This is a delicate surgical exercise requiring exact suturing methods and meticulous debridement without removal of skin.**

Surgical Procedure

General anesthesia is induced and maintained with the horse in lateral recumbency. The protective dressings should be removed and/or the contact lens removed, washed, and replaced. The wound is then irrigated with warm sterile saline, and sterile hydrogel applied to the wound site. To avoid further damage or hair contamination of the wound, the hair surrounding the wound should be clipped carefully.

The wound is then irrigated with sterile saline to remove all traces of the hydrogel, and all debris and foreign matter debrided with fine plain forceps, taking special care not to further damage any skin flap(s). The flap should be replaced into the natural position to keep it warm and clean. *No skin should be removed, no matter how damaged or non-viable it appears.*

The site is then prepared for aseptic surgery. If the orbital bone is damaged, small non-viable fragments should be removed and the orbital rim restored to a smooth outline. The wound site and the eye itself should be repeatedly irrigated with sterile warm saline delivered by a constant flow or by syringe during surgery.

A reassessment should then be performed, and reconstructive surgery planned in order to restore the functional eyelid. Accurate and careful assessment of the totality of structures involved is important. Palpebral conjunctiva is repaired with 0.7 metric (6/0) polyglactin so that no suture material is exposed on the inner surface of the conjunctival wound; exposed suture material may cause serious corneal damage. A conjunctival deficit can usually be reconstructed from adjacent loose conjunctiva. The relevant muscles should be accurately apposed using 1.5 metric (4/0) polyglactin, and a carefully placed suture of 0.7 metric (6/0) polyglactin inserted to ensure exact apposition of the eyelid margin. The knot should be drawn away from the eyelid margin itself. One end of the suture may be passed under the second suture and then tied again. In this way the marginal suture cannot impinge on the cornea. Alternatively, a modified figure-of-eight suture can be used (Figure 82).

If there is a skin deficit, a flap extension graft from the adjacent normal skin can be considered.

The skin incision is then closed from the palpebral margin outwards using 1.5 metric (4/0) polyglactin or monofilament nylon. Hydrogel should then be applied to the site of injury, and a stent made up of a gauze roll oversewn.

The stent is removed or replaced after 2 days; if the overlying sutures are tied suitably they can be untied to permit stent changes. An ice pack can be helpful in reducing swelling. Figure 82 shows the repair procedure for a full thickness lower eyelid laceration.

Eyelid Deficits

If there is a significant eyelid deficit the principles of management must include an accurate reconstruction of the eyelid so that the cornea is protected. Reconstructive surgery should be undertaken immediately, but if a delay is unavoidable the cornea must be protected by a bandage contact lens and continuous flow of artificial tears; this can be delivered via a subpalpebral lavage system with a dose balloon delivering 10 ml of artificial tears in 2–3 hours. Occasional topical application of artificial tears can be difficult in horses with painful eyelid damage.

Basic Principles of Reconstructive Eyelid Surgery

Normal eyelid tissue should be preserved as far as possible. Surgical reconstruction should be undertaken as soon as is practicable and aims to restore eyelid congruity and function. Up to 25% of loss can be compensated for by simple closure of the defect in the standard manner outlined above. Defects greater than 25% require reconstructive surgery.

Advancement flaps can be used to restore the eyelid but it is important to ensure full support for the flap by careful deep walking sutures. This will provide support and bulk for the eyelid. Restoration of the upper lid is much more difficult because of the complex muscular functions. There is usually no difficulty with deficits of conjunctiva as spare tissue is usually readily available.

No suture material should impinge on the cornea; if this is unavoidable a contact lens can provide corneal protection. The repaired eye must be protected from self-trauma by using a 'donut' bandage.

Follow-up Measures

The cornea should be examined daily (using fluorescein stain). As long as a contact lens is comfortable it can be left *in situ*. In any case the lens should be removed or replaced after 4–6 days, and can be removed after suture removal (7–10 days after surgery).

Antibiotics and non-steroidal anti-inflammatory drugs are normally used.

Ice packs can be used to keep swelling to a minimum following surgery.

If there is any eyelid distortion particular care must be taken to ensure that corneal damage/drying does not take place. Artificial tears (e.g. Viscotears; Ciba Vision) may be used prior to corrective surgery.

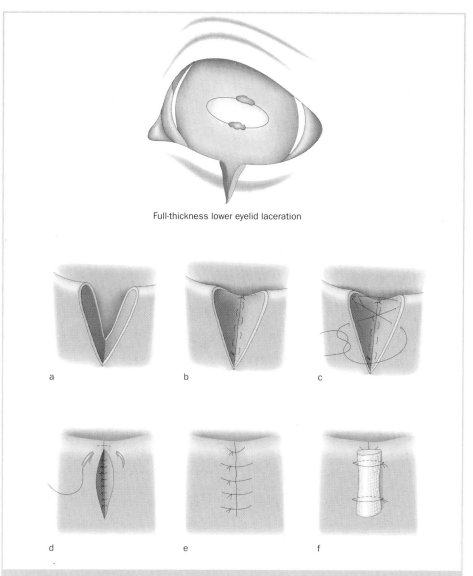

Full-thickness lower eyelid laceration

a

b

c

d

e

f

Figure 82a–f (a) The wound is carefully debrided without removal of skin. (b) The palpebral conjunctiva is closed using fine absorbable material in a continuous horizontal mattress suture pattern so that no suture material is exposed on the inner surface. (c) A figure-of-eight suture is laid to appose the eyelid margins. The knot will then lie away from the contact margin of the eyelid. (d) The subcutaneous tissues are closed and the skin is closed using simple interrupted sutures. (e) The closed wound should restore the integrity of the eyelid and its contact surface with the cornea. (f) A supportive stent fashioned out of cotton swab soaked in hydrogel or made from a conformable dressing is a useful way of protecting and supporting the wound site.

Eye Injuries

Introduction

Traumatic eye injuries are intolerant of delays or complications. The prognosis is inevitably poor with full thickness corneal laceration, or when there are complicating factors. If the injury also involves the lids or the medial/lateral canthus, the eye must be the primary concern. There is little point in treating an eyelid injury and leaving a serious corneal injury. Furthermore, attempts to examine the eye may result in irretrievable damage. Corneal injuries alone do not bleed significantly, but concurrent damage to the iris or the ciliary body may bleed heavily. Continued heavy bleeding is a poor prognostic sign. There are two types of corneal injury: *full thickness injuries* with total collapse of the anterior chamber (with or without lens luxation and collapse of the posterior chamber [vitreous leakage]) or with iris prolapse (usually with only partial collapse of the anterior chamber), and *partial thickness/flap injuries*.

Most full thickness corneal lacerations result in iris prolapse into the wound. This often limits aqueous humor loss and the drop in intraocular pressure. The prognosis of injuries where iris prolapse limits anterior chamber collapse is much better than those in with total collapse. There is a high rate of collateral intraocular damage. If the lens or the vitreous have been lost the prognosis for the eye is hopeless.

Full assessment allows rational treatment adjustment. A careful ultrasonographic examination (possibly under general anesthesia) may identify non-visible internal injuries. Partial or complete (anterior or posterior) lens dislocation can occur. Retinal detachment is a serious complication.

> ## Note
>
> **Horses with corneal injuries should be referred immediately to a specialist center, taking first aid steps before departure. The prognosis is usually poor with full thickness lacerations, but depends heavily on the delay to treatment, the extent, and the complications.**

Preliminary Approach

Examination can be facilitated by administration of an auriculopalpebral block. *No pressure should be applied to the eye, or the lids forced apart.* Heavy sedation or general anesthesia is preferred. The eye must be protected from further trauma, such as by using a protective 'donut' bandage (Figure 83).

Parenteral antibiotic is advised (penicillin is probably most useful), and topically applied antibiotic drops (gentamicin or choramphenicol is probably best) if this can be done without any pressure being applied to the eye. Parenteral non-steroidal anti-inflammatory drugs (e.g. telzenac, phenyl-butazone, or ketoprofen) and systemic opioid analgesics (e.g. butorphanol) are useful. If the horse is inclined to further self-trauma, sedation with an α-2 agonist (e.g. romifidine, detomidine, or xylazine) is helpful. The horse should then be moved to hospital (or referred to hospital).

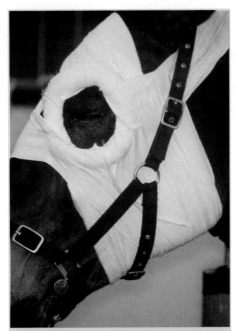

Figure 83 A 'donut' bandage used to protect an injured eye. An overlying protective pad can safely be applied to this dressing without risk of exacerbation of the injury.

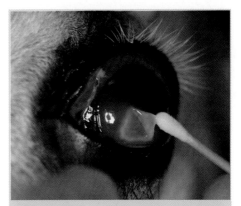

Figure 84 A partial corneal laceration. Fluorescein stain has been used to demonstrate the ulcer and the flap. The flap was surgically excised under standing sedation and topical anesthesia and the ulcer treated in routine fashion. There was no disability and no scar.

Note

Do not try to repair any full thickness corneal injuries under sedation or local anesthesia.

Surgical Procedure

The eye should be protected during induction of anesthesia, using a protective (induction) helmet or a large 'donut' bandage. The corneal surface is then flushed with warm sterile saline, and examined under a microscope to establish if there are secondary/concurrent injuries in the fundus (e.g. lens luxation, retinal detachment, and posterior chamber hemorrhage). Ultrasound scanning with a 10 mHz sector or 7.5 mHz linear scanner can be useful. Care must be taken not to apply any excessive pressure to the globe.

Partial Thickness Laceration (Figure 84)

The conjunctival sac is flushed with copious saline, and a very dilute povidone iodine solution (1 drop in 250 ml saline) can be used to flush the corneal surface.

111

Topical local anesthetic can then be applied. A decision needs to be taken as to whether the flap is to be removed or preserved.

Flap removal is used if the flap is shallow and non-viable. This can be performed under standing sedation and topical anesthesia (with auriculopalpebral motor block). Removal of the flap with corneal scissors placed obliquely ensures a close incision avoiding pocketing of the attached margin (Figure 85). The wound is then flushed with saline and treated as a shallow ulcer. A conjunctival flap graft may be placed, but this definitely requires general anesthesia so this decision needs to have been taken earlier! Antibiotic cover is provided by gentamicin drops applied every 2 hours (possibly using a sub-palpebral lavage system). Anti-collagenase medication such as EDTA, acetylcysteine, serum, or Galardin) can be given and topical corticosteroid used to limit scarring or fibrosis when there is negative fluorescein staining.

Flap restoration by suturing back into position is used when the flap is large, deep, and probably viable. It should not be used if the flap is non-viable or possibly infected or if there has been undue delay since injury. The horse is given a general anesthesthetic, and stay sutures and bridle sutures placed to stabilize the globe. The flap is then examined and irrigated thoroughly with warm sterile saline and antibiotic solution. The flap is replaced and sutured into position using 0.5 (8/0) polyglactin interrupted sutures (Figure 86). The injury is treated as a corneal ulcer until healed (see above), and then topical corticosteroids can be applied.

Full Thickness Laceration (Figures 87, 88)

General anesthesia and microscopic surgical facilities are compulsory. The periorbital skin should be clipped and prepared for aseptic surgery. A lateral canthotomy is performed if access to the injury is limited. Stay sutures and bridle sutures should be inserted to stabilize the eye and ensure good exposure.

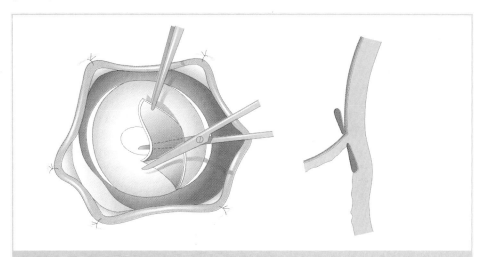

Figure 85 Diagram showing the technique for surgical excision of a non-viable superficial corneal flap. Note the placement of corneal scissors so that no pocketing is left at the attached margin. (Modified from JD Lavach, *Large Animal Ophthalmology* 1990, Mosby.)

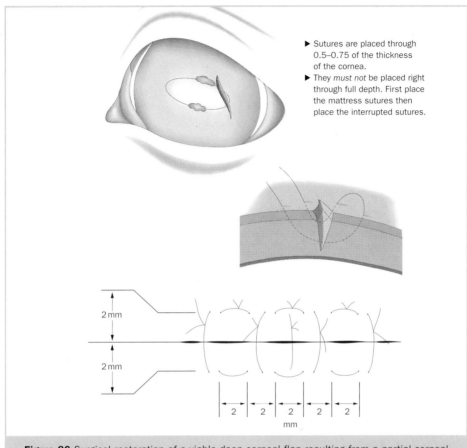

▶ Sutures are placed through
0.5–0.75 of the thickness
of the cornea.
▶ They *must not* be placed right
through full depth. First place
the mattress sutures then
place the interrupted sutures.

2 mm

2 mm

2   2   2   2   2
mm

Figure 86 Surgical restoration of a viable deep corneal flap resulting from a partial corneal laceration. (Modified from JD Lavach, *Large Animal Ophthalmology* 1990, Mosby.)

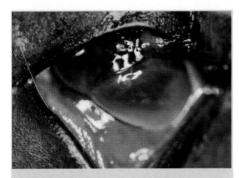

Figure 87 Full thickness corneal unjury. Because the injury was presented within minutes, repair was attempted.

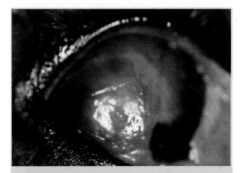

Figure 88 The consequent corneal fibrosis and internal damage resulted in negligible vision. Nevertheless, the eye was non-painful and cosmetically acceptable.

The full extent of the injury is then determined and if necessary hemorrhage controlled with adrenaline drops.

The margins of the laceration should be identified and carefully debrided, removing as little as possible of the corneal tissue without displacing the prolapsed iris. Interrupted horizontal mattress sutures of 0.5 (8/0) polyglactin should be placed (but not tied) from one side of the laceration to the other without disturbing the prolapsed iris tissue (Figure 89).

Sutures should penetrate up to two-thirds of the cornea only. Once all interrupted sutures are laid, the iris is either amputated (if non-viable or damaged or infected), or restored to the anterior chamber using a glass rod. The sutures are then tied sequentially towards the center of the wound. Simple interrupted sutures may then be placed between the mattress sutures. Large blood clots can be flushed from the anterior chamber before closing the wound.

It is useful to re-inflate the anterior chamber with sterile saline. A subpalpebral lavage system allows easy medication with antibiotics and anti-collagenase drugs every 2 hours for the first 5 days. Gentamicin drops, Viscotears and EDTA-plasma can be administered via the system. The lateral canthotomy is closed with 1.5 metric (4/0, USP) polyglactin, and the eye protected by a 'donut' bandage or helmet during recovery.

Systemic medication is essential. Antibiotics (penicillin/gentamicin) should be administered daily for 5–7 days, as intraocular infection is catastrophic. Non-steroidal analgesics (e.g. flunixin, phenylbutazone) are required to control pain and reflex/traumatic uveitis. Corneal sutures may be removed after 10 days but usually they decay spontaneously.

Follow-up Measures

Protection of the injured eye from further trauma is very important. A blepharoplasty to close the eyelids or a third eyelid flap to cover the cornea are sometimes used. However, these procedures will totally obscure the cornea and so it is difficult to assess progress. (Surgical procedures for these techniques are described in standard surgical texts.) 'Donut' dressings or face blinkers can be used to protect the eye while allowing assessment.

Corneal infection can be catastrophic, and so prevention of intraocular/superficial infection is paramount. Antibiotics and other medications that might be required, including atropine and artificial tears, can be delivered conveniently by use of a subpalpebral lavage system. Insertion of a system is described in standard surgical and ophthalmology texts, but the procedure is simple and effective.

In order to prevent corneal degeneration an anticollagenase solution (e.g. EDTA-plasma, acetylcysteine, or Gallardin) can be administered. An antibiotic/anticollagenase collyrium (Table 4) can provide the medication required. If these ingredients are not available then EDTA-plasma is a good alternative with topical antibiotics.

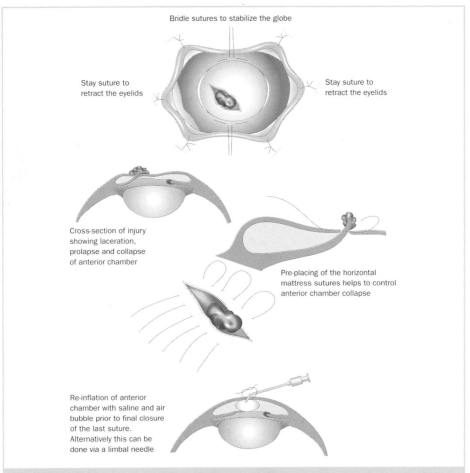

Bridle sutures to stabilize the globe

Stay suture to retract the eyelids

Stay suture to retract the eyelids

Cross-section of injury showing laceration, prolapse and collapse of anterior chamber

Pre-placing of the horizontal mattress sutures helps to control anterior chamber collapse

Re-inflation of anterior chamber with saline and air bubble prior to final closure of the last suture. Alternatively this can be done via a limbal needle

Figure 89 Surgical repair of a full thickness corneal laceration with iris prolapse. Note the preplaced mattress sutures make the process very much easier. (Modified from JD Lavach, *Large Animal Ophthalmology* 1990, Mosby.)

Table 4 Collyrium for topical therapy of corneal injuries

Infection type			
Gram negative		Gram positive	
Ingredient	Volume	Ingredient	Volume
Gentamicin (50 mg/ml)	5 ml	Chloramphenicol	8 ml
Atropine (2%)	5 ml	Atropine (2%)	10 ml
Acetylcysteine (20%)	15 ml	Acetylcysteine (20%)	15 ml
Artificial tears	5 ml	Artificial tears	10 ml

Wounds Involving the Mouth, Tongue, and Jaws

Introduction

Wounds involving the lips and mouth are important because they may prevent eating. Nevertheless, most horses are often seemingly unconcerned with minor or even some major lip/mouth/oral injuries. Blunt injury from kicks are frequently complicated by facial, mandibular, maxillary or orbital/zygomatic and cranial fractures, or eye or duct (salivary or nasolacrimal) injury. Lacerations to the tongue and the lips usually heal rapidly without significant scarring, unless there are complications. Maxillary and mandibular fractures and dental avulsions are relatively common in horses.

Preliminary Approach

The injury should be assessed carefully with a gloved finger (if necessary under sedation), and all the structures involved identified. Radiographs may be required. The eye must be examined in detail, and congruity of the jaws checked.

Dramatic injuries may be less significant than some minor ones. For example, a trivial facial injury from a kick might be complicated by a jaw or skull fracture. Damage to the skull may have serious implications: cranial fractures may be minor but have critical implications (see p. 119). Sinus depression fractures are common but seldom life threatening. Jaw fractures may appear disastrous but the prognosis is usually favorable. Hemorrhage should be controlled if possible. Sources of bleeding should be examined; bleeding from the ear or nose or hemorrhage into the fundus of the eye are serious signs.

Surgical Procedure

Skin wounds are packed with hydrogel, and the area clipped to reveal the full extent of the skin injury. Soft tissue injuries can be repaired under local analgesia using regional sensory blocks of the various sensory branches of the trigeminal nerve (infraorbital, frontal, or mental nerves). The area should be irrigated carefully with sterile saline and the wound debrided.

The affected soft tissues can then be repaired. Fractures and dental avulsions require special attention as soon as possible. Lip injuries must be repaired very carefully to avoid subsequent scarring and difficulty with eating. Mucosal injuries are usually left to heal by second intention.

Note

If there are complicating factors these should be dealt with as separate wounds (e.g. parotid duct, sinuses, teeth, and gingivae). Neurological signs suggestive of central nervous system injury should be managed carefully to reduce cerebral swelling/edema. Cranial fractures can be successfully managed in suitable hospital conditions but the horse may not be fit to travel. Surgical elevation of depression fractures is a rewarding procedure in horses. The wound can be closed by primary union after the reduction of any fractures and any other damage has been addressed.

Follow-up Measures

A soft diet may be indicated, although most horses will attempt to eat even when seriously injured. Routine antibiotics, analgesics and non-steroidal analgesics should be used. Sutures and fixators should be removed as soon as possible.

Scarring of the face and/or the oral structures can result in long-term disability and so scarring should be minimized by appropriate care with the healing process.

Wounds Involving Nerve Damage

Introduction

Injuries involving peripheral nerves are relatively common in the horse but seldom only involve the nerve itself (Figures 90, 91). Anatomical knowledge of the major (and important minor) nerve trunks is important. Nerve damage in wounds is usually serious and recovery is slow or commonly repair does not take place. The extent of the deficit and the exact location of the nerve as well as the functional type of nerve dictate the prognosis.

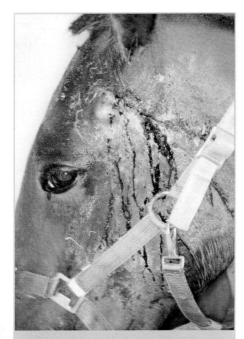

Figure 90 This gelding became trapped between two metal bars and lacerated itself in the left parotid region.

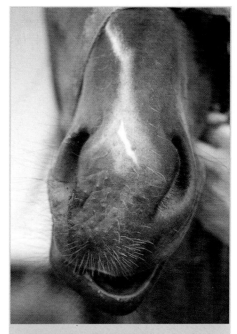

Figure 91 The laceration involved disseverance of the facial nerve with consequent permanent left facial paralysis.

Temporary damage is called neuropraxia while complete/permanent damage is called neurotmesis/axonotmesis. Nerve regeneration is very slow (approximately 0.5 cm per year). There are no practical ways yet available for repair of nerve injuries in horses.

Damage to nerves results in loss of sensation (if sensory nerve damage, when inadvertent subsequent self-trauma can occur), loss of motor function (loss of muscle function, weakness, and disability) or both sensory and motor function loss. Specific nerve trunks most commonly subjected to injury include:

Cranial nerves:
• Optic nerve.
• Facial nerve.
• Vestibular nerve.
• Hypoglossal/vagus and glossopharyngeal nerves within the guttural pouch may be damaged by fracture of the hyoid bone or the calvarium (pterygoid and sphenoidal fractures).

Peripheral nerves:
• Suprascapular nerve.
• Brachial plexus.
• Radial nerve.
• Femoral nerve.
• Sciatic nerve.
• Peroneal (fibular nerve).

Preliminary Approach

The full extent of the injury should be established, including a neurological damage assessment to identify all the structures involved. These should then be prioritized. Owners may not be unaware of the implications or signs of neurological compromise. Major nerve trunks usually run closely with major arteries and veins, e.g. the digital nerves run with digital arteries and veins in the neurovascular bundles. For this reason bleeding should be controlled by direct pressure *only*, as a clamp could be inadvertently applied to the nerve, causing serious problems.

In a few cases the nerve can be sutured. Most minor injuries to nerves have temporary neuropraxia, and recover spontaneously over some weeks or months.

Pain control and support for the type of injury involved are important. Complete loss/absence of pain is possible if the nerves are badly damaged, but this is not reliable and should not preclude the necessity for local analgesia. The horse should not be moved if it appears unable to bear weight (this usually means that the motor nerves are damaged or there may be fracture involvement).

Surgical Procedure

Hydrogel should be applied to the wound prior to preliminary clipping and irrigation. The damaged tissues should be identified and treated accordingly (see other sections). The damaged nerve must be protected from any further damage.

Repairing the nerve by realigning the severed ends and suturing the nerve sheath with 0.7 metric polyglactin can be attempt under general anesthesia but is seldom feasible.

Follow-up Measures

Rehabilitation of horses with motor deficits can be very slow and requires sustained physiotherapy. Secondary trauma can arise from motor deficits: for instance, facial nerve trauma causes difficulty with eating and/or paralysis of the upper eyelid, which can cause serious corneal degeneration.

The prognosis for traumatic nerve injuries is complicated by neuroma formation in some cases. The nerve may be hyperesthetic or even show extreme pain or may envelope the adjacent blood vessels with consequent distal ischemia.

Wounds Involving Cranial Damage

Introduction

Cranial injury is frequently fatal either immediately or soon after the injury. Fracture of the cranium is invariably involved. The extent of injury may belie its severity. Euthanasia is usually indicated but there are reports of recovery even from severe damage.

Preliminary Approach

Sedation and even general anesthesia may be required. Most affected horses are unconscious or show severe neurological deficits (bizarre behavior, seizures, or profound depression/stupor/coma). Exposed brain tissue must be kept moist with saline throughout the period of assessment.

Heavy systemic corticosteroids and non-steroidal anti-inflammatory drugs are usually administered to reduce inflammation/edema related damage. Diuresis with intravenous mannitol may reduce or at least limit the swelling. Intracranial bleeding can be a serious complication.

Surgical Procedure

Under general anesthesia the skin wound is opened and any loose bone fragments are removed, if necessary from the brain tissue. All obviously damaged brain tissue is removed. The meninges are reconstructed to provide a protective barrier for the wound site. The skin is reconstructed after the cranium is restored to its best possible position.

Follow-up Measures

Recovery from anesthesia is often problematical, and it is sometimes necessary to keep the horse heavily sedated or even anesthetized for 24–36 hours after surgery. Ponies and foals are easier to manage and so carry a slightly better prognosis. *Undue suffering must be prevented*, and so the large majority of cases result in euthanasia and so a very serious initial decision should be made.

Wounds Involving Hoof Capsule and Coronary Band

Introduction

The hoof is susceptible to injuries in the form of lacerations, abrasions, contusions, and penetrations. Healing of hoof injuries is invariably slow and difficult. Secondary injuries from weak or damaged horn (e.g. wall break-back, avulsion, or laceration) may heal with a permanent scar or deformity. Injuries involving the coronary band will usually result in a permanent hoof defect. This may be significant or clinically unimportant, but will usually involve remedial farriery to some extent (Figures 92–94).

Preliminary Approach

It is important to establish the involvement of deeper structures such as synovial cavities, neurovascular tissues, bones (PII, PIII, navicular), collateral cartilages, and digital cushion. The extent of hoof capsule damage must be determined, including the involvement of germinal epithelium (particularly in the coronary band), the presence of contaminant material under the remaining hoof capsule, and the degree of resultant hoof capsule instability, and the viability of the damaged tissues should be established.

Radiography is advisable to check for injuries to the phalanges and navicular bone, and to search for radiodense foreign bodies.

Surgical Procedure

Control of hemorrhage and removal of the worst of the contaminants should be performed. Hydrogel should be applied, and any obvious cavity filled with a conforming sponge dressing, or conforming non-felting swab with hydrogel.

The area should be clipped (and/or rasped) and the surrounding epidermis prepared, by carefully inspecting the horn around the margins of the wound, and removing the hoof wall overlying contaminated tissues.

The totality of structures involved should be assessed; this may involve intra-synovial injection to check for joint capsule trauma/penetration. If this is present, the management of the wound will be complicated by the need to flush and repair the joint/sheath involved (see p. 100). All contaminated and non-viable tissue must be removed.

Sterile dressings with a moist wound environment are applied, ensuring that dressings are impervious from the outside (e.g. by the use of adhesive nylon tape). Natural and 'chemical' debridement (e.g. using Intrasite Gel plus Allevyn Cavity) is maintained until the wound appears free of infection.

Decisions must be made whether to apply a rigid limb cast (either with secondary or delayed primary intention healing), to apply a supportive shoe to stabilize the hoof capsule through surgical farriery or a repair to the hoof defect with synthetic resin, or to use repeated bandaging with regular examination (usually second intention healing).

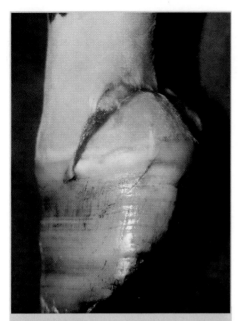

Figure 92 This young colt suffered severe wire lacerations involving the coronary band over a short distance.

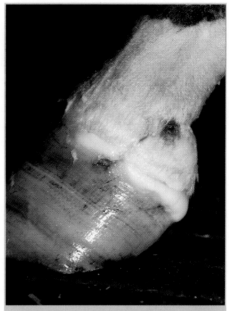

Figure 93 The wound in Figure 77 was handled very carefully with removal of foreign matter, and healed well. There remained an obvious horn defect with a scar at the coronet.

Figure 94 A severe laceration involving avulsion of a large portion of the coronary band and hoof wall. The injury was treated with the aid of a rigid limb cast. Extensive hoof wall deficits remained, but the mare remained pain free and mobile. (Courtesy of RR Pascoe.)

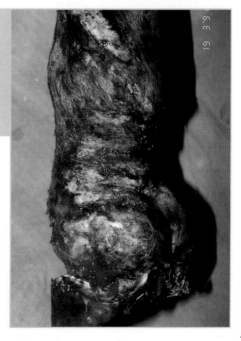

Follow-up Measures

Injuries involving the coronary band almost inevitably result in a permanent hoof defect. Complications and defects can be minimized by thorough wound management and dedicated farriery. The prognosis for injuries involving deeper structures depends on early recognition of complications and speedy, effective treatment.

Wounds Involving Open Body Cavities

Introduction

Wounds that involve the body cavities are always critical. Thoracic wounds that open the chest result in aspiration of air into the pleural cavity. Injuries that also damage the visceral pleura (and therefore puncture the lung) allow air to fill the pleural cavity. They are commonly complicated by fractured ribs that may also puncture the lung.

Abdominal wounds that open the peritoneal cavity are not often immediately life threatening. However, prolapse of abdominal viscera (gut, spleen, or omentum are commonest) are critical, and require emergency attention. Injuries that result in severe contamination of the chest cavity or the peritoneum (or abdominal viscera) carry a very poor prognosis. The cause of the injury may have considerable implications.

Chest injuries are for the most part probably more significant immediately than abdominal injuries, because of the consequent pneumothorax. Abnormal fast shallow breathing patterns are associated with lung collapse. Mucous membranes may be cyanotic and congested. The two pleural cavities may not be contiguous and so it is important to assess both lungs and to use radiographs if these are available. It may be possible to hear air being sucked into the wound during inspiration. Horses with severe pneumothorax (with lung collapse and/or intrathoracic hemorrhage) may be very distressed and the signs may be mistaken for colic. The horse may be reluctant to move due to parietal (pleural) thoracic pain, and any movement may exacerbate the distress and the severity of the respiratory embarrassment.

Abdominal injuries are possibly more common than chest injuries. There may be little distress in the first instance in spite of herniation or pneumo-peritoneum.

Herniation of abdominal viscera is a very serious complication because of the risks of (ongoing) damage to the structure and because of possible infection. Herniation of intestine is the commonest complication of abdominal wounds.

If peritonitis (with parietal pain) is present then the horse will likely be reluctant to move and may 'guard its abdomen'. Guarding can be detected by trying to press on the belly wall just below the costochondral arch. As pressure is applied, the horse will tense the abdominal musculature. It may show significant pain when the pressure is released and it may 'grunt'. Horses with significant peritonitis will also be febrile, and there will be a high white cell count and total protein in the peritoneal fluid. The extent and the viability of the herniated intestine give a good indication of the prognosis. Large lengths of severely damaged and compromised bowel carry a poor or hopeless prognosis.

Penetrating foreign bodies such as farm implement tines or wooden or metal fence posts cause some abdominal injuries, and there may be leakage of ingesta into the peritoneal cavity. This caries a poor or hopeless prognosis unless by chance the damage is restricted to a small accessible area.

> ## Note
>
> **Injuries to the chest and abdominal walls that penetrate into the respective cavities, which are over 12 hours in duration may be irretrievably infected by multiple bacteria (including Gram negative organisms and anaerobes).**

Preliminary Approach

The horse must be restrained, and stress and excitement minimized by quiet handling. In some cases the animal may be very distressed, but if the chest is affected very serious thought should be given before sedation is used. For abdominal injuries (with prolapsed viscera) sedation can usually be safely given without difficulty. The metabolic and clinical status should be assessed with particular attention to the respiratory tract if the chest is involved. It is likely that injuries in these categories will require surgery so food should be withheld.

Chest Injuries

Respiratory function should be checked by auscultation and by careful clinical assessment. If air can be heard moving in and out of the wound site, a clean dry dressing should be placed over the site and held in place so that more air cannot be sucked in. Sucking of air on inspiration is the more dangerous sign suggestive of lung collapse.

Penetrating objects should not be removed from the wound unless and until there are suitable measures available to control/prevent a pneumothorax. The wound should not be washed until it is cleaned as far as possible; washing will merely mean that bacteria and foreign matter are easily sucked into the chest. It may be possible to pack the wound with a sterile gel or with a saline soaked swab until the area has been clipped and disinfected.

The wound site should be examined by careful digital palpation (simultaneous auscultation over the site might confirm crepitus if a rib is fractured). The wound site should be covered with hydrogel on a pad, or a conformable dressing used to occlude the wound site. The area can then be carefully clipped, and cleaned as carefully as possible. Introduction of soluble antibiotic (e.g. crystalline penicillin and gentamicin combination) into the chest is advisable; if metronidazole injection is available then this should be introduced immediately also.

Abdominal Injuries

The prolapsed viscera will seldom be returnable to the abdomen and in any case this should not be done without thought and care. It is likely that surgery will be needed, so the prolapsed tissues should be cleaned and protected from further damage. If the defect is large enough to restore the gut safely to the abdomen, then it may be replaced after careful saline washing and removal of all foreign matter. For the most part, wounds on the ventral abdomen that have intestinal herniation are not amenable to any sort of immediate repair.

Any prolapsed tissues should be supported by a saline soaked cotton or nylon sheet and lifted up to the abdomen: this will prevent the structures being damaged and will reduce the tension on blood vessels. It will also prevent further contamination or infection. Copious warm saline should be poured over the sheet to keep it moist while the horse is moved to a surgical facility.

Surgical Procedure

Chest Injuries

If possible, the muscles, subcutis, and skin are closed in separate layers. If it is not possible to close the wound it should be covered with a stent and a bandage around the chest (Elastoplast is suitable). Fractured ribs are commonly involved and all loose pieces of bone should be removed. It may be very difficult to close either the pleura or the overlying muscles if ribs have been damaged and removed, or if the ribs fail to provide support for the wound closure. *The horse should be referred immediately to a specialist center or admitted to hospital.*

Note

There is a major risk of septic pleuritis, and thoracic lavage with antibiotics is urgently required.

Abdominal Injuries

All exposed viscera must be protected throughout the preparation for surgery.

The wound area is protected from contamination during preparation by hydrogels and copious saline lavage. The viability of the herniated tissues will have a profound effect on the management of the case.

Once the visceral problems have been addressed, the abdominal wound should be managed as for lacerations. Closure of the wound is essential except in exceptional circumstances when other means may have to be employed.

The various layers of abdominal musculature or aponeuroses must be identified and closed in multiple layers where appropriate. The peritoneal cavity will almost invariably be infected and inflamed, and so copious peritoneal irrigation during (and possibly after surgery) may be indicated.

Placement of a peritoneal drain is a useful way of removing exudate, and transabdominal flushing can be used either via a dorsally placed ingress portal or directly via the peritoneal drain. Antibiotics can be administered directly via the lavage solution and/or systemically.

Follow-up Measures

In both thoracic and abdominal injuries there is a very serious risk of infection. Strong and prolonged antibiotic therapy is always indicated. Thoracic or peritoneal drains should be maintained until the inflammation and exudate has become manageable. Recovery may take a very long time (up to 12 months or more), and the rate of postinjury complication (usually from adhesions or chronic infection) is high.

Wounds Involving Major Blood Vessels

Introduction

Damage to blood vessels is an inevitable consequence of all skin injuries. In spite of severe damage to large vessels, horses very seldom bleed to death as a result of blood vessel laceration. Bleeding eventually stops even in moderate arterial blood loss circumstances. The major neck arteries and veins are probably the most dangerous in this respect. The vessels involved dictate the clinical signs and the likely consequences.

In areas that have large or well-developed collateral circulation, damage has less clinical significance than areas where the vessels are anatomically restricted. For example, damage to the palmar digital arteries in the pastern or metacarpal regions may deprive large ipsilateral areas of the foot of blood supply. By contrast, damage to superficial vessels on the skin of the trunk usually can be compensated for by collateral circulation. Spiral wounds may involve both the medial and lateral palmar (plantar) digital vessels and so the foot is totally deprived of blood supply.

Comparison of the surface temperature below the injury, particularly the foot, with that of the other limbs will help to assess the extent of vascular impairment.

Damage to blood vessels is often accompanied by damage to the sensory nerves because they commonly run together (see p. 117). The type of vessels damaged also has important clinical implications: arterial damage results in high pressure bleeding and it may be more difficult to control the bleeding both naturally and by therapeutic measures; venous bleeding is usually slow and, unless there are complicating factors such as blood clotting disorders, bleeding usually stops relatively quickly. Capillary bleeding is usually insignificant in horses.

Cessation of bleeding from all types of vessel relies heavily on clotting (coagulation). It is usually possible to assess clotting directly from the wound site or the blood on the floor. Hemophilia is rare in horses (usually seen only in foals). Acquired hemorrhagic diatheses include liver failure, disseminated intravascular coagulopathy (DIC), and drug related bleeding, including warfarin (used for treatment of navicular syndrome) and aspirin (sometimes used either to control cataract development or as an anti-inflammatory, antipyretic analgesic).

Preliminary Approach

Blood loss should be controlled immediately. Direct pressure is usually sufficient for most purposes. Larger arterial bleeding may require ligation (but particular care must be taken to identify correctly the bleeding artery alone). Pressure bandages are useful, but can cause serious damage if incorrectly applied and left in place for too long.

Swabs with adrenaline can be used to cause profound vasoconstriction in difficult sites (e.g. wounds involving the cornea and sclera). Dressings should not be removed until there are other methods for controlling any bleeding. Wounds that bleed heavily should probably not be washed or flushed in case the clot is displaced and bleeding recurs. However, secondary bleeding is seldom critical in equine wounds. An alternative means of controlling bleeding should be ready when flushing takes place.

Surgical Procedure

The wound must be thoroughly cleaned and any identifiable foreign body removed. This frequently entails excision of connective tissue and other grossly contaminated or damaged tissues using a scalpel and dissecting forceps. Extensive debridement of this nature is often best performed under general anesthesia.

The advantage gained from the provision of optimum surgical conditions far outweighs the risks and difficulties of getting the horse to a suitable surgical facility. Bleeding arteries can be ligated but there is a risk in some anatomical sites of distal total ischemia if this is done. Anastomosis of severed arteries is seldom performed in horses, but may be applicable to distal limb lacerations.

Problems can arise when the bleeding vessels cannot be identified or are located deep in the wound (e.g. eye, brain, chest, mouth, or nasal cavity injuries). Direct pressure may be impossible to apply either because of lack of access or because pressure itself causes significant damage. In this case, alginate dressings can be helpful. Diathermy or laser coagulation can also be helpful.

Follow-up Measures

Particular care must be taken to make regular assessments of the blood supply to the tissues distal to a damaged artery. Venous and capillary bleeding are seldom of any major concern even when relatively large veins are involved, or in the case of capillaries, large areas of tissue are involved.

10 The Future of Wound Management

Since 1962 there has been a major revolution in the understanding of wound healing as a physiological process. However, the research has inevitably focused on the laboratory animal, and the clinical bias has been towards the human species. The particular problems faced by horses in their tendency to wounding and their known difficulties with healing, have not been addressed seriously until the last 5 years.

Management of the acute wound in horses is clearly a critical factor; immediate intensive management of a wound can make a vast difference to the way in which it heals. The once highly regarded 'golden period' in which bacteria were present but not in a replicative adherent fashion, was used to emphasize the importance of early intervention in the management process of wounds. Now the same philosophy is applied to more diverse aspects of wound care. It is now clear that the fastest healing occurs when the inflammatory process is rapid, intense, and transient. The manner by which ponies heal so well in contrast to larger horses suggested that it was worth examining the healing processes in a comparative way. In the future there may well be ways of enhancing the 'sluggish' acute inflammatory response characteristic of larger horses, and allowing it to terminate rapidly, so that the wounds will more accurately follow the healing process of ponies. This will be a major advance but in reality it is likely to be far more complicated than just applying a dressing that contains high concentrations of TGF-beta! The complex interrelationships that exist between the various growth factors means that all efforts have to be directed towards reducing any harmful effects as far as possible. In this way we at least try to encourage the normal healing process. Of course, given the remarkably efficient healing in ponies, it is easy to view the problems in larger horses as the result of man's interference in breeding larger horses! Therefore there may be a future in genetic studies of the wound healing process, and the inflammatory response in particular.

The particular problems the horse suffers, particularly in respect of the notoriously bad healing capacity of the healing process of the distal limb regions of the larger horses (over 145 cm), has continued to frustrate the clinician. In a few cases healing proceeds uneventfully (just as it does on the body trunk of horses and the limb and trunk of ponies less than 145 cm), but in others the wounds not only fail to heal but actually expand. Exuberant granulation tissue is a really serious issue in horses that has at last come under direct scrutiny. In the first instance the clinician needs to eliminate any of the overt causes of failure of wound healing, and having completed this should use the best possible dressings to ensure a rapid repair. The faster the repair, the less the opportunity for exuberant granulation tissue or the development of an indolent wound or abnormal scarring.

Wound dressings are an area where there has been much progress. Historically, wound dressings were regarded as a passive aspect of wound management. They were almost all made from various forms of cotton (lint, cotton, wool, gauze swabs) and were designed to cover and conceal the wound. A major role was in hiding exudates and sealing in the unpleasant smells and purulent exudates that were typically present. Many older dressings had positively harmful effects on wound healing (e.g. wet–dry dressings), and fortunately these have lost any relevance in modern wound management. The concept of moist wound management proposed in 1962[10] changed the whole philosophy, so that dressings were then regarded as being an active part of the management of wounds. From a position where wound management products formed a very small part of the medical and veterinary pharmacopoeias in the middle of the 20th century, there are now thousands of products, each being advertised with amazing reports of instant solutions to wound problems. The reality is however, that this large armamentarium of products simply provides the clinician with opportunities to select appropriate dressings for each stage of each individual wound. There is even now no single dressing that is applicable to all stages of all wounds, and indeed no wound that can be managed simply by a single universal dressing.

In human wound care scar management is a major factor. There are several reasons for this including the obvious cosmetic advantages. Scarring in humans can be a major limiting factor in restoring normal function because wound contraction can be extremely powerful and persistent. Fortunately in horses, scarring is seldom problematical apart from the cosmetic aspects in show horses. In some sites however, such as the cornea, scarring can limit function and so scar management is a significant aspect of wound care.

The future of wound management is being driven by clinical need and by the creditable desire to restore the horse to normal as soon as possible. There are welfare and commercial forces that will gradually advance our understanding of wound management. New wound care products (dressings and hydrogels in particular) are being developed in response to the improving awareness that it is possible to improve healing dramatically by correct selection of the best products for particular circumstances. Only through clinical research and commercial cooperation will we find enough resource to solve the many aspects of wound care that remain.

References

1   Wilmink JM, Stolk PWT, Van Weeren PR, and Barneveld A. Differences in second intention wound healing between horses and ponies: macroscopical aspects. *Equine Vet J* 1999; **31**:53–60.

2   Wilmink JM, Van Weeren PR, Stolk PWT, *et al*. Differences in second intention wound healing between horses and ponies: Histological aspects. *Equine Vet J* 1999; **31**:61–67.

3   Wilmink JM, Nederbragt H, van Weeren PR, *et al. Differences in wound contraction between horses and ponies are not caused by inherent contraction capacity of fibroblasts*. PhD Thesis, University of Utrecht, Netherlands 2000; 85–100.

4   Desmouliere A, Geinoz A, Gabbiani F, and Gabbiani G. Transforming growth factor-β1 induces a smooth muscle actin expression in granulation tissue myofibroblasts and in quiescent and growing cultured fibroblasts. *J Cell Biol* 1993; **122**:103–111.

5   Lanning DA, Nwomeh BC, Montante SJ, *et al*. TGF-β 1 alters the healing of cutaneous fetal excisional wounds. *J Pediatr Surg* 1999; **34**:695–700.

6   Hackett RP. Delayed wound closure, a review and report on the use of the technique on three equine limb wounds. *Vet Surg* 1983; **12**:48.

7   Stashak TS. Skin grafting in horses. *Vet Clues of Nth Am* 1984; **6**:215.

8   Knottenbelt DC. Equine Wound Management: Are there significant differences in healing at different sites on the body? *Vet Dermatol* 1997; **8**:273–290.

9   Pascoe RR, and Knottenbelt DC. *Manual of Equine Dermatology*. London: WB Saunders; 1999.

10 Winter GD. Formation of the scab and the rate of epithelialization of superficial wounds in the skin of the young domestic pig. *Nature* 1962; **93**:293–294.

11 Gamgee S. Absorbent and medicated surgical dressings. *Lancet* 1890; **1**:127.

12 Wilmink, JM. Wound Healing in Horses: *The role of inflammation and contraction*. PhD Thesis, University of Utrecht, Netherlands 2000; 148–150.

13 Pascoe RR, and Knottenbelt DC. *Manual of Equine Dermatology*. London: WB Saunders; 1999.

14 Lees MJ, *et al*. Principles of skin grafting. Compendium for Continuing Education I989; **11(8)**:954–960.

15 Rogers BO. Historical development of skin grafting. *Surg Clin North Am* 1959; **39**:289–311.

16 Wilmink JM. Modified Meek Technique for the management of chronic non-healing wounds in horses. *Proc Vet Wound Healing Assoc*: Annual Scientific Meeting, Hanover, Germany, May 2001.

17 Lees MJ *et al*. Tunnel grafting of equine wounds. *Compendium for Continuing Education* 1989; **11(8)**:962–969.

18 Swaim SF. Principles of mesh skin grafting. *Compendium of Continuing Education* 1982; **4(3)**:194–202.

19 Diehl M, and Ersek PA. Porcine xenografts for treatment of skin defects in horses. *J Am Vet Med Assoc* 1990; **177**:625–628.

20 Shah M, Foreman DM, and Ferguson MJW. Neutralising antibody to TGF-β reduces cutaneous scarring in adult rodents. *J Cell Sci* 1994; **107**:1137–1157.

Index